INDOOR ROWING

Your Complete Guide to Training, Programming, and Workouts

Caley Crawford, NASM-CPT
Michelle Parolini, NASM-CPT

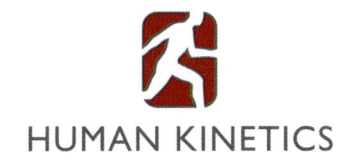

HUMAN KINETICS

Library of Congress Cataloging-in-Publication Data

Names: Crawford, Caley, 1989- author. | Parolini, Michelle, 1970- author.
Title: Indoor rowing : your complete guide to training, programming, and workouts / Caley Crawford, NASM-CPT, Michelle Parolini, NASM-CPT.
Description: Champaign, IL : Human Kinetics, [2025] | Includes bibliographical references.
Identifiers: LCCN 2024025113 (print) | LCCN 2024025114 (ebook) | ISBN 9781718226593 (paperback) | ISBN 9781718226609 (epub) | ISBN 9781718226616 (pdf)
Subjects: LCSH: Indoor rowing--Training.
Classification: LCC GV543.2 .C73 2025 (print) | LCC GV543.2 (ebook) | DDC 613.7/16--dc23/eng/20240712
LC record available at https://lccn.loc.gov/2024025113
LC ebook record available at https://lccn.loc.gov/2024025114

ISBN: 978-1-7182-2659-3 (print)

Copyright © 2025 by Caley Crawford and Michelle Parolini

Human Kinetics supports copyright. Copyright fuels scientific and artistic endeavor, encourages authors to create new works, and promotes free speech. Thank you for buying an authorized edition of this work and for complying with copyright laws by not reproducing, scanning, or distributing any part of it in any form without written permission from the publisher. You are supporting authors and allowing Human Kinetics to continue to publish works that increase the knowledge, enhance the performance, and improve the lives of people all over the world.

To report suspected copyright infringement of content published by Human Kinetics, contact us at **permissions@hkusa.com**. To request permission to legally reuse content published by Human Kinetics, please refer to the information at **https://US.HumanKinetics.com/pages/permissions-translations-faqs**.

This publication is written and published to provide accurate and authoritative information relevant to the subject matter presented. It is published and sold with the understanding that the author and publisher are not engaged in rendering legal, medical, or other professional services by reason of their authorship or publication of this work. If medical or other expert assistance is required, the services of a competent professional person should be sought.

The web addresses cited in this text were current as of April 2024, unless otherwise noted.

Senior Acquisitions Editor: Michelle Earle; **Developmental Editor:** Amy Stahl; **Managing Editor:** Kim Kaufman; **Copyeditor:** Joan Little, Pendulum Editing; **Permissions Manager:** Laurel Mitchell; **Graphic Designer:** Dawn Sills; **Cover Designer:** Keri Evans; **Cover Design Specialist:** Susan Rothermel Allen; **Photographs (cover and interior):** Kirk Fitzek/© Human Kinetics, unless otherwise noted; **Photo Asset Manager:** Laura Fitch; **Photo Production Specialist:** Amy M. Rose; **Photo Production Manager:** Jason Allen; **Senior Art Manager:** Kelly Hendren; **Illustrations:** © Human Kinetics; **Printer:** Versa Press

We thank The Bar in Irvine, California, for assistance in providing the location for the photo shoot for this book.

Human Kinetics books are available at special discounts for bulk purchase. Special editions or book excerpts can also be created to specification. For details, contact the Special Sales Manager at Human Kinetics.

Printed in the United States of America   10 9 8 7 6 5 4 3 2 1

The paper in this book is certified under a sustainable forestry program.

Human Kinetics	*United States and International*	*Canada*
1607 N. Market Street	Website: **US.HumanKinetics.com**	Website: **Canada.HumanKinetics.com**
Champaign, IL 61820	Email: info@hkusa.com	Email: info@hkcanada.com
USA	Phone: 1-800-747-4457	

E9335

INDOOR ROWING

Your Complete Guide to Training, Programming, and Workouts

CONTENTS

Drill, Exercise, and Workout Finder vii
Preface xi
Introduction xiii

PART I ROW FOR LIFE

1 WHY ROW? 3

2 UNDERSTAND THE ROWER 15

PART II LEARN PROPER ROWING

3 ROWING TECHNIQUE 29

4 COMMON ERRORS IN ROWING 41

PART III SAMPLE ROWING WORKOUTS AND STRETCHES

5 TYPES OF WORKOUTS 63

6 WARM-UP AND COOL-DOWN 71

7 ENDURANCE WORKOUTS 109

8 INTERVAL WORKOUTS 115

PART IV **CUSTOMIZE YOUR PROGRAM**

9 OFF-THE-ROWER STRENGTH TRAINING FOR ON-THE-ROWER PERFORMANCE 123

10 INCORPORATING ROWING INTO STRENGTH AND FITNESS ROUTINES 149

11 SAMPLE SIX-WEEK ROWING PROGRAM 157

References   187
About the Authors   189
Earn Continuing Education Credits/Units   192

DRILL, EXERCISE, AND WORKOUT FINDER

Chapter 4: Common Errors in Rowing

Body Over Pause and Double Pause Drills	43
Catch Hold Drill	56
Heavy Handle Drill	51
Legs Only Pick Drill	46
Low Stroke Rate Drill	58
Strapless Rowing Drill	53

Chapter 6: Warm-Up and Cool-Down

Arms Only Pick Drill	96
Bird Dog	79
Cat–Cow	78
Child's Pose	80
Dowel Rod–Assisted Good Mornings	74
Dynamic Half Pigeon	94
Good Mornings	75
Hand Release Push-Ups	86
High Plank to Downward Dog	82
Hip Rotation	91
Inchworms	85
Legs Only Pick Drill	98
Power Stroke Warm-Up	102
PVC or Banded Shoulder Pass Throughs	81
Reverse Lunge	87
Sphinx T-Spine Rotation	83
Squat Stretch	89
Standing Hip Cradle	84

Steady-State Rowing as a Warm-Up	100
Stroke Rate Ladder as a Warm-Up	100
Tin Soldier	88
Walkout + Push-Up	90
Walkouts	76
World's Greatest Stretch	92

Cool-Downs

Cobra Stretch	107
Downward Dog + Hip Shifts and Foot Pedals	106
Half Pigeon Static Stretch	104
Runners Lunge + Arm Reach	105

Chapter 7: Endurance Workouts

Endurance Workout #1: 8,500-Meter Stroke Rate Ladder	110
Endurance Workout #2: Steady Repeat	111
Endurance Workout #3: Descending 6,000-Meter Row	113

Chapter 8: Interval Workouts

1:1 Work-to-Rest Ratio	118
10 Minutes of Vanishing Intervals	118
15-Minute Power Stroke EMOM (Every Minute on the Minute)	118
Tabata Blast: 2:1 Work-to-Rest Ratio	118

Chapter 9: Off-the-Rower Strength Training

Gluteus

Barbell Hip Thrust	125
Split Squat	126

Hamstrings

Romanian Deadlift (Strength)	127
Towel Hamstrings Stretch (Flexibility)	128

Quadriceps

Jump Squat	131
Skater Jump	132

Core

Medicine Ball Slams (Strength)	134
Suitcase March (Stabilization)	133

Latissimus Dorsi

Bent-Over Row	135
Dumbbell Pullover	136

Pectoral Muscles

Chest Press	138
Push-Ups	140

Shoulders

Overhead Press	141
Upright Row	142

Triceps

Lying Triceps Extension	143
Triceps Dips	144

Spinal Erector Muscles

Good Mornings	146
Superman	145

Chapter 11: Sample Six-Week Rowing Program

Week 1, Workout 1	158
Week 1, Workout 2	160
Week 1, Workout 3	162
Week 2, Workout 1	164
Week 2, Workout 2	166
Week 3, Workout 1	168
Week 3, Workout 2	170
Week 4, Workout 1	172
Week 4, Workout 2	174
Week 4, Workout 3	176
Week 5, Workout 1	178
Week 5, Workout 2	180
Week 6, Workout 1	182
Week 6, Workout 2	184

PREFACE

We have been an integral part of an indoor rowing-based fitness franchise since its very beginning and have trained thousands of unique individuals, with rowing as the primary focus of the workouts. The primary benefits of indoor rowing include improved cardiorespiratory (cardio) health and full-body exercise with low impact and low risk of injury. These benefits bring in a wide variety of clientele, including many people who haven't worked out in years or ever before. When rowing properly, anyone can gain results that are comparable, if not superior, to other forms of cardio training. In fact, rowing is a full-body exercise that has a strength component, so some might find it superior in benefits to other exercises like cycling or running. This book will get anyone feeling more confident, powerful, and capable in their rowing execution.

Having had the opportunity to witness the impact this modality of fitness has had on so many people, we have seen how special indoor rowing is. Rowing is often the best fitness solution for so many people and can be an exercise done for life. It is also very clear to us that although many people have previously experienced rowing in a fitness environment, they have never learned correct form and therefore cannot maximize their benefits and results from the machine. As the rowing machine becomes more renowned as an efficient and effective form of exercise, a need exists for education on the benefits of rowing, the mechanics behind the rowing stroke, and the common misconceptions of indoor rowing and how to overcome them. This book will provide a roadmap to help demystify the modality and offer a clear path for anyone interested in using the machine as a vehicle to their ultimate health.

The book's structure provides a progressive path to learning this unique modality and movement pattern.

Part I gives readers a quick snapshot of the sport's longevity and the types of rowing machines on the market. From there, we dive into part II and the mechanics of the stroke! When used properly, the rowing machine works the majority of the muscles in the body, far more than other cardio machines in the gym. Other common cardio choices, like running and cycling, have familiar movement patterns that people have usually perfected over time. Rowing, on the other hand, does not have this familiarity. Typical leisure activities like kayaking and canoeing are the rowing activities with which people are familiar. Both use primarily the upper body. This results in the common misconception that rowing is an upper-body-focused movement, when in fact your legs and core generate roughly 90% of the power in your stroke. We'll provide an outline of how special populations can modify the rowing stroke or the machine setup to accommodate any fitness level and most injuries or restrictions.

Parts III and IV provide direction on how to build safe, effective, and comprehensive workouts based on goals. Rowing is fantastic for both interval and endurance training, providing both muscular and cardiorespiratory conditioning. Understanding the difference between the energy systems used and how the rower taps into each is critical to developing a well-rounded workout. Conditioning off the rower is also important, as is finding ways to incorporate floor-work strength training into the rowing workout to build strength on and off the rower. In addition to providing direction on program design, this book includes 21 workouts, complete with post-rowing stretching routines for personal training, group fitness, and individual program design.

INTRODUCTION

Though there are discrepancies among scholars regarding when rowing races began, rowing as a mode of transportation began before 1500 BC (Koch 2018). Ancient Egyptian artifacts illustrate people rowing or paddling on a boat with an oar or a paddle. A wall etching even shows a crew of people rowing, seated, with oars in hand. This specific artifact dates from 1507 to 1458 BC and even shows the oars and oarlocks on the boat's side. Oarlocks are small hooks or enclosures that hold the oar and provide a pivot point while taking strokes. Using oarlocks is one of the key differences between paddling and rowing, and it is believed that paddling came before rowing because oarlocks were a later development.

Rowing as a sport began in England in the late 17th and early 18th centuries. The first collegiate men's race was between Oxford and Cambridge in 1829. Rowing gained popularity and traveled to America in the 19th century, becoming the country's first intercollegiate sport. Every year, there are major collegiate regattas or races in the United Kingdom, Australia, the United States, and Canada. Rowing has been a part of every Olympic Games (except 1896 in Athens), with women's rowing debuting in the 1976 Montreal Olympics.

Rowing's unique characteristic is its need for camaraderie and synchronicity for the boat to move far and fast. A variety of boat sizes are raced: singles, doubles, quads, or 8-person. Regardless of the boat's size, people remember the athletes working together as a whole, not a specific athlete. Each seat in the boat has a specific purpose, and they must work together to propel it forward. The more in sync they are, the faster the boat moves. This is called swing, and it's unique to the sport.

In rowing, a boat is also called a *shell*. When *sweep rowing*, athletes hold one oar in their hands. Athletes most commonly perform sweep rowing in a pair (with or without a *coxswain*, or the person steering and coaching the boat), a four (with or without a coxswain), or an eight (with a coxswain). When *sculling*, athletes hold two oars in their hands. Athletes most commonly perform sculling as a single, a double, or a quad.

Rowing has been around for thousands of years, but it is now getting the attention it deserves as an "off-the-water" fitness modality. It is one of the most underutilized and under-instructed forms of exercise for the general population and fitness professionals alike. Rowing engages most of the muscles in the body, including the glutei, hamstrings, quadriceps, and calves in the legs; the latissimus dorsi, trapezius, and rhomboids in the back; all the core muscles, including the erector spinae; and the shoulders, biceps, and triceps in the arms. And rowing uses the most important muscle of all—the heart muscle!

Roles and Responsibilities of Each Seat in the Boat

Rowing is the one sport that you move forward by looking back! All of the rowers are facing in the opposite direction of the movement of the boat. The coxswain steers the boat and coaches the athletes on the water. In rowing, athletes are defined by their seat in the boat (see figure I.1). The seats begin with the bow, which is the part of the boat that crosses the finish line first. From there, the seat numbers move from 2 to 7, ending with seat 8, which is the *stroke seat*. The stroke seat must be a strong technical rower with excellent consistency in their stroke because the other athletes in the boat follow their cadence, or stroke rate. Thought of as the *stroke's lieutenant*, seat 7 helps hold the tempo and cadence of the stroke because it's directly behind the stroke seat. Seats 7 and 8 are the *stern pair*. Seats 4, 5, and 6 are the *engine room*, which is typically where the strongest and most powerful athletes sit to build momentum and speed. Coaches often put their least technical rower in seat 3 because they believe this seat has the least impact on the boat's performance. Seats 1 and 2 are the *bow pair*. Their role is to balance the boat. Each seat serves a unique purpose and contributes to the overall speed and success of the boat in a race or regatta.

Sculling Boats

Single (1x):
One rower, no coxswain

Pair (2-):
Two rowers with one oar each

Double (2x):
Two rowers with two oars, no coxswain

Four (4+):
Four rowers with one oar each with or without coxswain

Quad (4x):
Four rowers with two oars each, with or without coxswain

Eight (8+):
Eight rowers with one oar each with coxswain

FIGURE I.1 There are various types of boats in the sport of rowing. While the boats may seem similar, each one is unique and requires a different skill set from the athletes. C = coxswain.

Rowing embodies the power that the human body can achieve through good body awareness, kinesthesia, and connection. Rowing provides a platform for both aerobic and anaerobic conditioning, as well as muscular conditioning and strength. According to a publication by the Harvard Medical School (2021), 30 minutes of vigorous rowing can burn from 255 to 440 calories, all done in a low-impact environment.

PART I

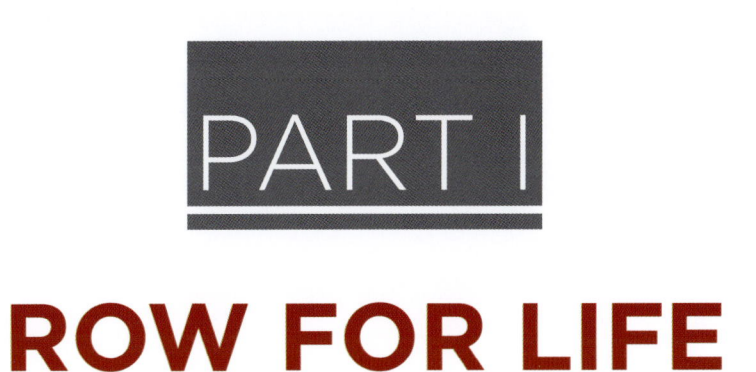

ROW FOR LIFE

1

WHY ROW?

There are many benefits to all forms of exercise; however, rowing's benefits supersede most other forms' by providing longevity for your body and overall wellness. In addition to the unique individual benefits of rowing, the compounded impact of those advantages truly sets rowing apart from other forms of exercise. In this chapter, we'll explore the many ways that rowing for exercise positively affects our fitness and our daily lives. Let's start by breaking them down into three main categories: cardiorespiratory benefits, muscular and joint benefits, and benefits that enhance activities of daily living.

Cardiorespiratory Benefits

Rowing is a highly effective cardiorespiratory exercise that improves the function of your heart and lungs. Some cardiorespiratory gains from rowing include the following:

- *Increased oxygen intake:* Rowing involves the continuous movement of large muscle groups in the body. A 2020 article by VO2 Master states that "muscles performing work require increasing amounts of energy as the workload increases, which correspondingly requires more and more oxygen." As a result, rowing will increase your oxygen intake because of the large recruitment of muscles, which will help to improve your overall lung capacity and cardiorespiratory health.

- *Improved energy and stamina:* Many rowing workouts require you to sustain a steady pace for an extended period, which can help to improve your endurance and stamina. This can translate to improved performance in other areas of your life, such as sports or other physical activities.

- *Lowered blood pressure:* Studies have shown that regular aerobic exercise can help to lower blood pressure (University of Colorado Hospital 2003; Mayo Clinic Staff 2024; Corliss 2021). Many doctors recommend exercise as a first-line treatment for high blood pressure (University of Colorado Hospital 2003; Mayo Clinic Staff 2024).

- *Increased calorie burn:* By engaging all the major muscle groups, rowing increases overall strength and cardiorespiratory capacity with one machine. Rowing can boost weight loss by providing a significant calorie burn. According to a publication by the Harvard Medical School (2021), 30 minutes of vigorous rowing can burn 255 to 440 calories, while 30 minutes of moderate-intensity rowing can burn 210 to 294 calories. The number of calories burned varies based on exercise intensity, which the user controls. Rowing can help to maintain a healthy weight, which is an important factor in reducing the risk of heart disease.
- *Improved cholesterol levels:* Cardiorespiratory (aerobic) exercise, like rowing, can help to reduce levels of LDL (bad) cholesterol in the blood, which is a major risk factor for heart disease (University of Colorado Hospital 2003).
- *Enhanced circulation:* Aerobic exercise, like rowing, increases blood flow throughout the body, which helps to enhance circulation and improve overall cardiorespiratory health (Johns Hopkins Medicine, n.d.a).
- *Lowered resting heart rate:* Regular aerobic exercise lowers your resting heart rate. Once you begin a rowing routine, you can expect your resting heart rate to lower. The large muscles used in the rowing stroke cause your heart to work harder and become more efficient. Your heart's stroke volume should also increase, delivering more oxygen and nutrients to the body's tissues and organs with each beat. As a result, the heart beats less each minute, which is reflected in a lowered resting heart rate (Chertoff 2023).
- *Improved heart rate recovery:* When rowing or exercising consistently, you can expect to see improved heart rate recovery (Cleveland Clinic 2022). If you review a graph of your heart rate during your workout, you can expect to see stronger peaks and valleys on the graph. Translated to daily life, you'll recover quickly and become less breathless when you walk up stairs, play with your dog, or chase a toddler.

Overall, rowing is an excellent form of cardiorespiratory exercise that can provide numerous benefits for your heart, lungs, and overall health. Whether you are a beginner or an experienced athlete, rowing can be a highly effective and rewarding addition to your fitness routine.

Muscular and Joint Benefits

Rowing is an excellent full-body exercise that engages muscles throughout the body, setting it apart from other cardiorespiratory exercise options. In chapter 3, we'll dive a little deeper into the specific muscles used in the movements of rowing. Figure 1.1 shows the amount of muscle you can activate in the rowing stroke when you're truly rowing well.

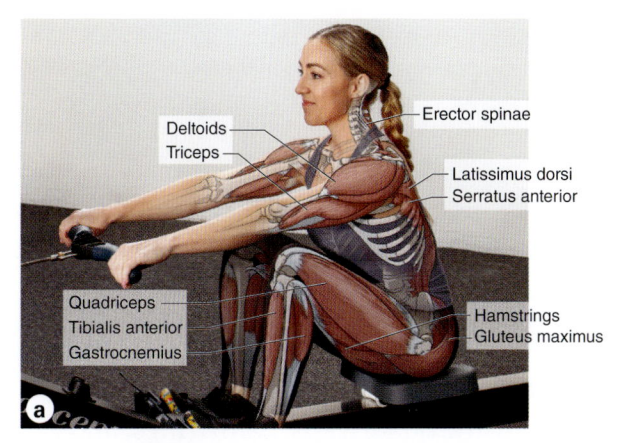

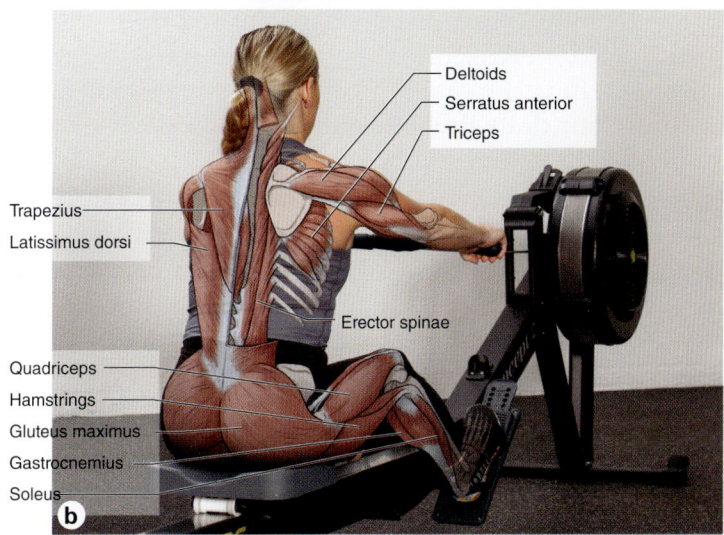

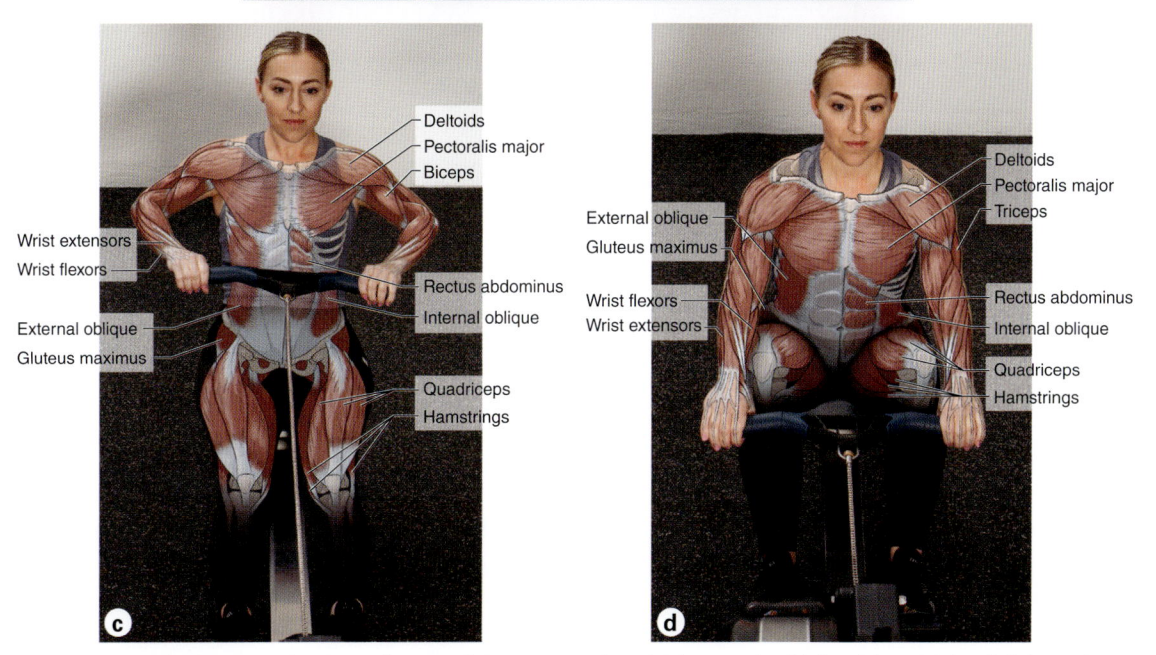

FIGURE 1.1 Active muscles in each part of the row stroke: *(a)* the catch, *(b)* the drive, *(c)* the finish, and *(d)* the recovery.

Consider some of the more specific muscular benefits.

- *Increased core strength:* Rowing engages major and minor core muscles, including the transverse abdominis, multifidus, internal and external obliques, erector spinae, diaphragm, and rectus abdominis. Your minor core muscles include your latissimus dorsi (lats), trapezius (traps), and glutei (glutes). A strong core is essential for maintaining proper posture, balance, and stability during everyday activities.

- *Increased lower body strength:* Rowing works the major muscles in your legs, including the quadriceps, hamstrings, and glutes. When applying force to the machine, these muscles contract and produce power and resistance, leading to increased leg strength and muscle development. Using and strengthening the major leg muscles supports healthy movement throughout your daily life, like climbing stairs, getting up from a chair, or simply bending your knees.

- *Increased functional strength:* Functional exercise is important because it focuses on movements and activities that are relevant to everyday life rather than simply targeting individual muscles in isolation. Rowing's movement pattern is incredibly functional in that it is easily replicated when picking something up and putting something down. By incorporating movements that mimic real-world activities, functional exercise can help to improve balance, coordination, flexibility, and strength in a way that translates to improved performance in daily life.

- *Improved posture:* By working the core, lats, and back muscles, rowing will strengthen the upper back and the musculature that supports the lumbar spine, which can result in improved postural alignment.

- *Triple joint extension:* Rowing is a triple extension movement, which means your ankles, knees, and hips will move through extension (and flexion) in every stroke. Mobility in these joints is crucial for aging bodies as well as for anyone recovering from an injury. The American Sports & Fitness Association (n.d.) states, "Older adults who remain flexible have a lower risk of falls and injuries. Flexibility also helps to maintain independence by allowing you to continue doing activities important to your quality of life, such as gardening or cooking. Being flexible also helps you avoid injuries and strains. If you are less flexible, it is more likely that your muscles will be put under greater strain when performing tasks such as lifting heavy objects or bending down, which increases the likelihood of injury."

- *Low impact:* One of the primary benefits of rowing as a form of exercise is its low-impact nature. Unlike running or other high-impact exercises, rowing is gentle on the joints and can be a great option for those who may be prone to injury or discomfort with other forms of exercise. Low-impact exercise reduces the risk of musculoskeletal injury caused by impact movement, making it a good option for people of all shapes, sizes, and fitness levels.

- *No weight bearing:* Rowing is a non-weight-bearing exercise, which means you're not bearing your body weight when exercising. This is important for anyone who's recovering from a lower body injury or is overweight because it creates less pressure on your joints. The rowing workout's low-impact and non-weight-bearing nature allows your body to recover quickly, which ultimately means you can row more in a shorter period, resulting in greater benefits.

Overall, rowing is an excellent exercise for building muscular strength and improving cardiorespiratory health. It engages a wide range of muscles in the body, making it a highly effective full-body workout. Now, it is important to note that because rowing is effort based, if you're not rowing properly or not producing any intensity or power on the machine, then you may not experience optimum results. It's important to learn and practice the proper rowing form so you can recruit the right muscles and begin reaping the benefits of this full-body exercise. Let's take a quick look at how variations in body position may load the muscles differently.

> **KEY POINT**
>
> It's important to learn and practice the proper rowing form so you can recruit the right muscles and begin reaping the benefits of this full-body exercise.

In figure 1.2*a*, the back is rounded. Pushing back in this position will likely put excess pressure on the back because of improper loading of the legs and core. In figure 1.2*b*, the spine is tall and the upper body is hinged forward to about 11 o'clock. This may not seem like a big difference, but in photo *b*, the hamstrings and glutes are loaded, the core is activated and braced, and the body is ready to take on a strong load. This athlete is likely to produce more power on the machine and, without a doubt, have more muscle activation.

Remember, when we activate and work more of our larger muscles, our heart grows stronger, the muscles grow stronger, and our workout is optimized. We'll dive into more on correct rowing form in chapter 3 so you can ensure you're rowing properly to get the most benefit from your rowing workouts.

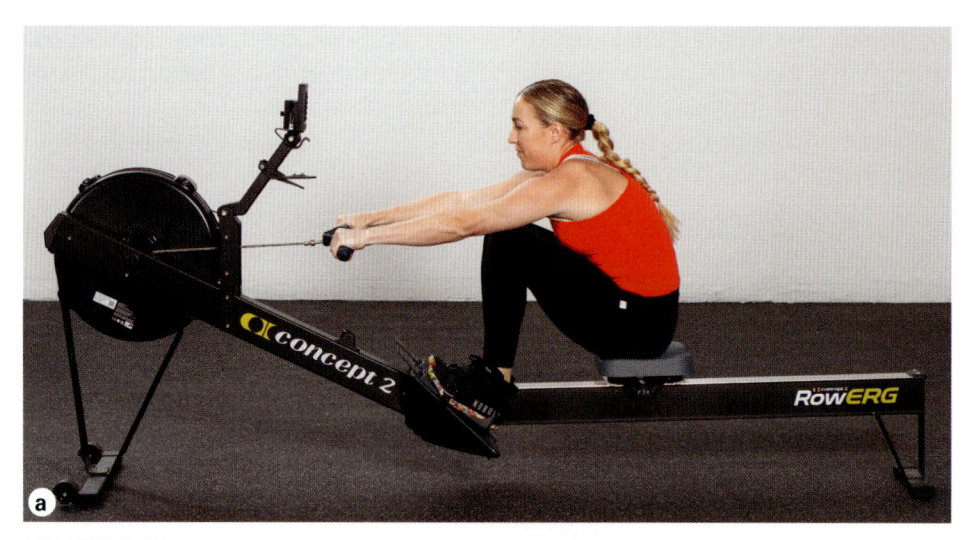

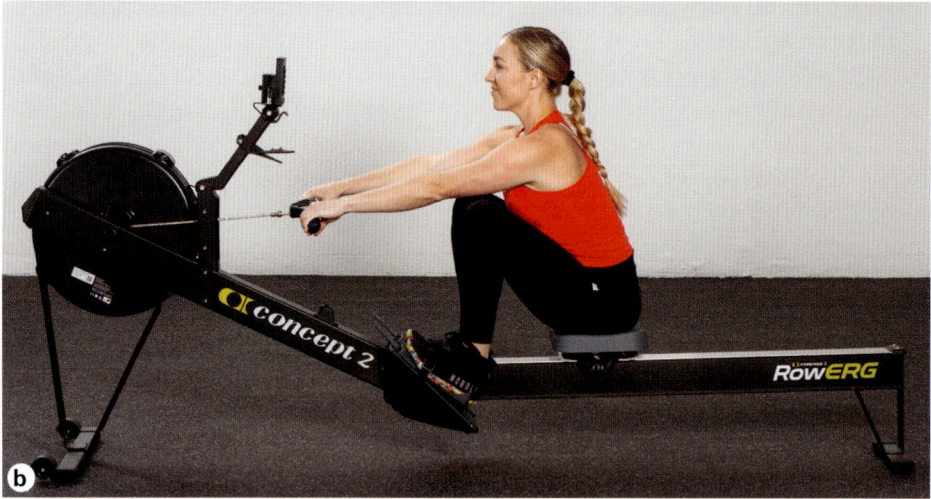

FIGURE 1.2 *(a)* Improper rowing stroke posture with a rounded spine and *(b)* proper rowing stroke posture with a strong, tall spine.

Benefits That Enhance Activities of Daily Living

The functional movement pattern of rowing translates to the movements we do in everyday life. Many say that rowing is a sport for life because the movement teaches your body's muscles to work together, similar to how we need them to function in daily life. Figure 1.3 illustrates how the motions you practice while rowing can help train you to more easily and efficiently perform everyday activities.

Why Row? 9

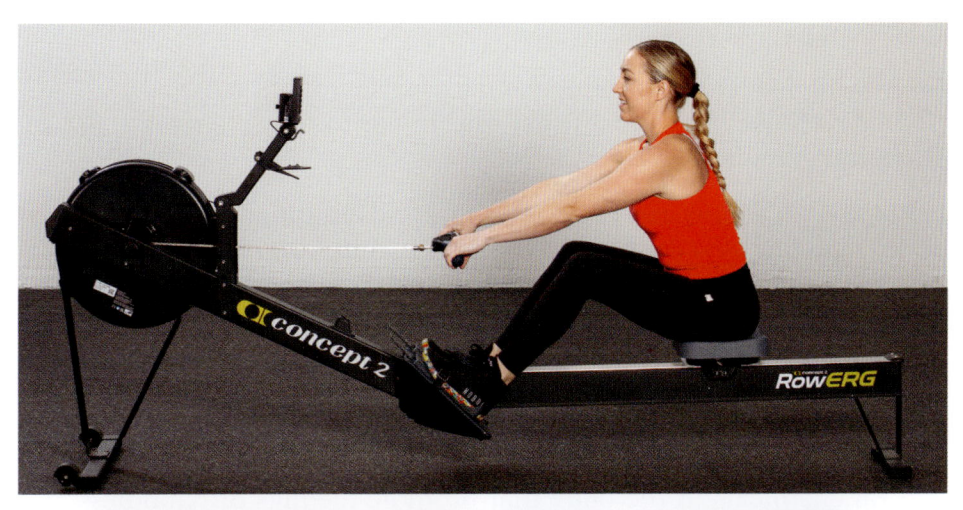

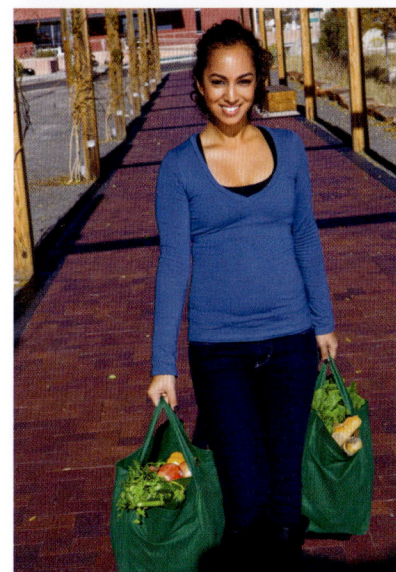

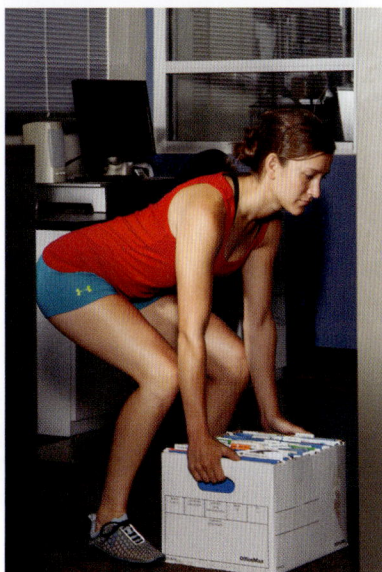

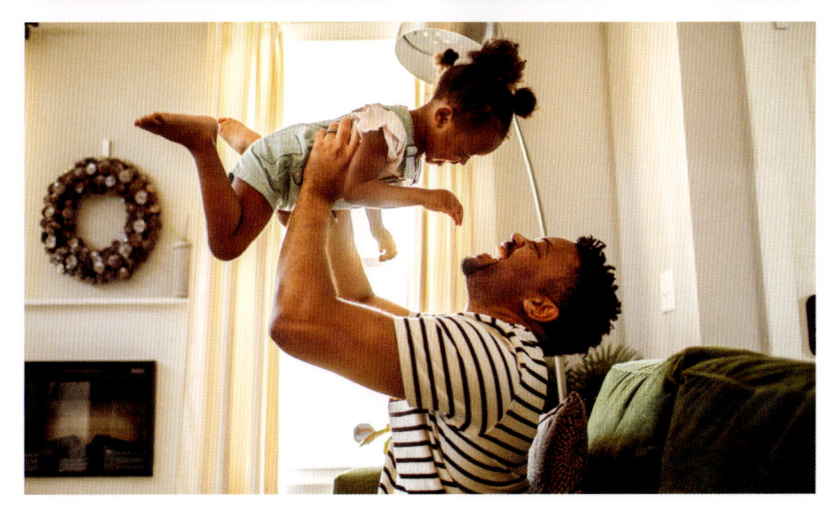

FIGURE 1.3 The rowing stroke helps you more efficiently perform your daily living activities.

> **KEY POINT**
> Rowing is a sport for life because the movement teaches your body's muscles to work together, similar to how we need them to function in daily life.

Rowing for fitness can provide mental and emotional benefits, as well as physical ones. By reducing stress and anxiety, improving mental clarity, increasing self-confidence, and improving sleep, rowing can help you achieve a greater sense of overall well-being and an improved quality of life. Rowing for your workout includes some of the following mental and emotional benefits:

- *Reduced stress and anxiety:* Cardiorespiratory exercise, like rowing, can help to reduce stress and anxiety by releasing endorphins, which are natural chemicals in the body that promote feelings of happiness and well-being. This can help to improve your mood and reduce feelings of stress and anxiety.
- *Improved mental clarity:* Regular cardiorespiratory exercise can help to improve mental clarity and focus by increasing blood flow to the brain and boosting cognitive function. This can help you feel more alert and focused throughout the day. Rowing is effort based, which means the user creates their intensity, resulting in strong mental focus and control.
- *Increased self-confidence:* Regular exercise can help to improve your self-confidence as you achieve your fitness goals and feel better about your health. This can lead to improved self-esteem and a more positive self-image.
- *Better sleep:* Cardiorespiratory exercise, like rowing, can improve your sleep by helping you fall asleep faster and stay asleep longer. This may improve your overall mood and energy levels throughout the day.

Rowing for Special Populations

Rowing is a sport for everyone. The rowing machine, also known as the *erg* (short for *ergometer*), is low-impact, making it accessible for those who may need special consideration when designing and following an exercise program. Special populations include older adults and those who have a medical or physical condition or possibly have a transient (temporary) medical condition like pregnancy or perimenopause. We'll look at four special population groups here: older adults, peri- and postmenopausal women, pregnant women, and postpartum women.

Older Adults

As we age, we are continually looking for ways to stay strong, mobile, and moving. Castillo-Garzón and colleagues (2006) state, "Appropriately undertaken, physical exercise is the best means currently available for delaying and preventing the consequences of aging, and of improving health and wellbeing." As we age, several physiological changes happen that can cause us to slow down or even move differently. It's important to note that aging is individual and is different from person to person. Factors such as lifestyle, genetics, and environment play a significant role in how aging affects each individual.

Some notable areas of the body that undergo changes over time are the bones, joints, and muscles. After age 35, bone breakdown occurs faster than bone buildup, which can result in a gradual loss of bone mass. For those with osteoporosis, loss of bone mass occurs at an even greater rate and can accelerate further after menopause. A loss of bone mass in the vertebral column and muscle mass loss in the supporting muscles can cause a person's overall height to shrink. Understanding how to row with good posture will not only increase the level of output on the rower, but it will also help keep the spine moving well and reduce bone and muscle compression.

Changes in the cardiovascular system as we mature may cause the heart to become less efficient at pumping blood to working muscles. Arteries become less elastic, leading to increased stiffness and thicker capillary walls. This may cause a slight increase in blood pressure. Proper warm-ups and cool-downs are essential for all older adults. Paying attention to how different movements impact your heart rate will allow you to select and develop the right training plan for you.

Diminished proprioception and balance are two factors typically associated with age. *Proprioception* refers to your understanding of where your body is in space. Why is proprioception important? Proprioceptors in tendons, muscles, ligaments, and joint capsules all work together to give feedback to the body so that it can work efficiently (Ferlinc et al. 2019). As our bodies age and those connections don't work quite as well, decreased proprioception affects everything from balance to ease of movement. Rowing can help increase our levels of proprioception by challenging us to perform the proper stroke pattern of legs, body, then arms on the drive and arms, body, then legs on the recovery. This heightened awareness of our movement not only works to strengthen those connections, but it can also bring about lower split times and more production on the machine.

Older athletes should consider the changes in joints and tendons that come with age, which can result in reduced flexibility and an increased risk of injury. Rowing is a low-impact form of movement that allows for full range of motion (triple flexion at the catch into triple extension at the finish) and lubrication of the joints with every stroke. Allow for longer warm-ups and cool-downs, and be OK with where you are in this stage of your life! We're aiming for longevity and overall health maintenance. Rowing provides a good mix of aerobics, strength and flexibility, and accessibility for all fitness levels.

Perimenopause and Menopause

Perimenopause can be described as the time when a female's ovaries gradually stop working (Johns Hopkins University n.d.b), which is a precursor to menopause. Common physical symptoms of perimenopause caused by changing hormone levels include hot flashes, difficulty sleeping, headaches and migraines, muscle aches and joint pain, and changes in metabolism and body shape. Symptoms can last for months or years and change over time.

Menopause occurs when you stop menstruating and go through 12 consecutive months without a period. Your doctor can take a blood sample to check hormone levels and confirm the onset of menopause. Postmenopause can create a host of issues, including cardiovascular disease, osteoporosis, moodiness, anxiety, and depression, brought about by hormonal and physiological changes.

Consistent cardiorespiratory exercise and strength training, coupled with stretching and meditation, can greatly improve how you go through this phase of your life. Rowing can help manage weight and maintain muscle, especially in the legs. Regular physical activity can combat the bone loss that occurs as a result of menopause. That same physical activity will act as a mood booster by releasing endorphins and keeping your heart healthy! Finally, staying active seems to have a positive impact on the frequency and intensity of hot flashes.

Pregnancy

Rowing can be a great form of exercise during pregnancy due to its low-impact and non-weight-bearing cardiorespiratory benefits. As suggested with any form of exercise while pregnant, it's important to check with your doctor to ensure exercise is safe. All pregnancies are different, and you may encounter unique circumstances that will or will not allow you to continue exercising.

Two considerations for rowing while pregnant are making sure that you have the proper form and that you understand how to adjust your intensity throughout your workouts. As the second and third trimesters come, the level of intensity that your body will be capable of will drop. The beauty of rowing is that it is effort based and easily adjusted with each stroke. A good rule of thumb is to perform a "talk test" throughout your workouts. The talk test simply allows you to ensure you're able to talk throughout your rowing efforts, which will help to maintain your intensity at a safe level.

Postpartum Considerations

Rowing can be an effective part of a postpartum exercise routine. Like rowing while pregnant, it's important to get clearance from your doctor before starting any exercise routine postpartum. Depending on whether you had a cesarean birth or a natural birth, your timeline for returning to exercise will differ. Typically, women who give birth via c-section will have a slightly longer timeline due to the time required to recover from surgery.

While rowing is a fantastic form of exercise for pre- and postpartum bodies, one factor to consider as you're ramping up is the core component of the exercise. Especially for women who have undergone a cesarean birth, the abdominal muscles will take some time to rebuild. The best approach to rowing postpartum, regardless of the type of birth, is to slowly increase the intensity and volume over time. It's important to start slow and listen to your body as best you can. Layering rowing into your postpartum routine has the benefit of strengthening your abdominals and improving your core connection very quickly. Rowing's low-impact and non-weight-bearing nature will help you ramp up your exercise without risking wear and tear on the body and joints. As always, form will be a very important component as you look to incorporate rowing into your pre- and postpartum exercise routines.

Rowing may not be the favorite workout for all people, but it works well for many. One of the key factors in gaining significant benefits and results from rowing is proper form, which we'll discuss more in chapter 3. Improving your body mechanics and timing in your rowing stroke can make a huge difference in your ability to get results. Rowing is effort based, so as you begin to learn how to activate more muscles in the stroke due to better body positioning, you'll enhance your ability to generate power on the drive. Before we get to how to improve your form, chapter 2 helps you understand the rowing machine itself so you can feel confident on the machine, whether it's your first or thousandth workout!

2

UNDERSTAND THE ROWER

At first glance, the rowing machine might strike fear in some people. The intimidation factor quickly dissolves when you learn how to use the machine and understand the multitude of benefits you get from this full-body workout. The rowing machine, also known as the *erg*, consists of a slide, a moving seat, and a handle attached to the resistance (air, water, or magnet).

Body mechanics on the rowing machine are critical for optimal muscle engagement. Learning how to use the erg correctly starts with learning what the specific machine you are using can do for you. Every rowing machine is unique, but all rowers deliver a workout that will give you both cardio and strength!

Types of Rowing Machines

Different types of rowing machines may have variations in their operation and functionality. Understanding the specific type of rowing machine you have allows you to use it correctly, ensuring that you derive maximum benefit from your workouts and avoid any potential safety risks. You may find that your split times from one type of machine to the next are not comparable based on the drive mechanism differences.

Some rowing machines come with preprogrammed workouts or different resistance settings and features that are specific to their type. By understanding the type of rowing machine you have, you can take advantage of these features and tailor your workouts accordingly. This allows you to set specific goals, track your progress, and optimize your training routine for better results.

In this chapter, we'll run through some of the most popular rowing machines, including hydraulic, water, air, and magnetic rowers. Figure 2.1 identifies the main parts of a rowing machine.

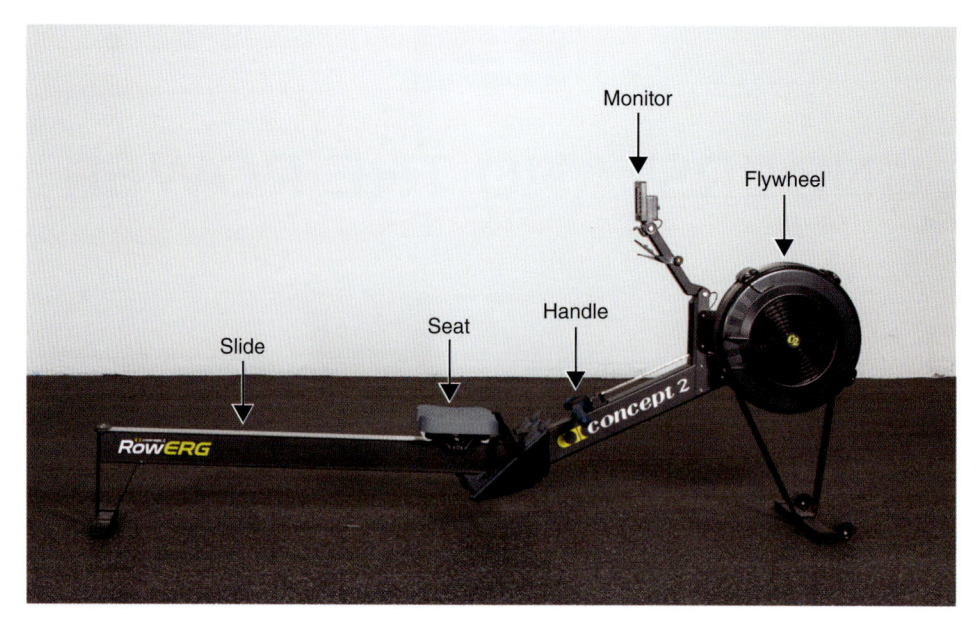

FIGURE 2.1 Anatomy of the rowing machine.

Hydraulic Rower

The hydraulic rower has a hydraulic resistance system consisting of two hydraulic pistons connected to the rowing handle. As the user pulls the handle toward their chest, the pistons compress and provide resistance, which creates the feeling of rowing against water. The resistance can be adjusted by changing the amount of fluid (oil or water) in the pistons or by adjusting the resistance setting on the machine.

Hydraulic rowers are popular for home use because they are relatively compact, easy to store, and tend to be quieter than other machines. Some drawbacks of the hydraulic rower are that it may not offer the same level of resistance or consistency in resistance as other types of rowing machines, such as air or water resistance rowers. However, if you're looking for something compact and inexpensive, the hydraulic rower will fit the bill!

Water Rower

The water rower (see figure 2.2) uses water to create resistance with a paddle that spins inside a water tank. This style of rower strives to provide an experience for the user that replicates the feel of the natural, on-water rowing stroke. The high density of water allows for continued

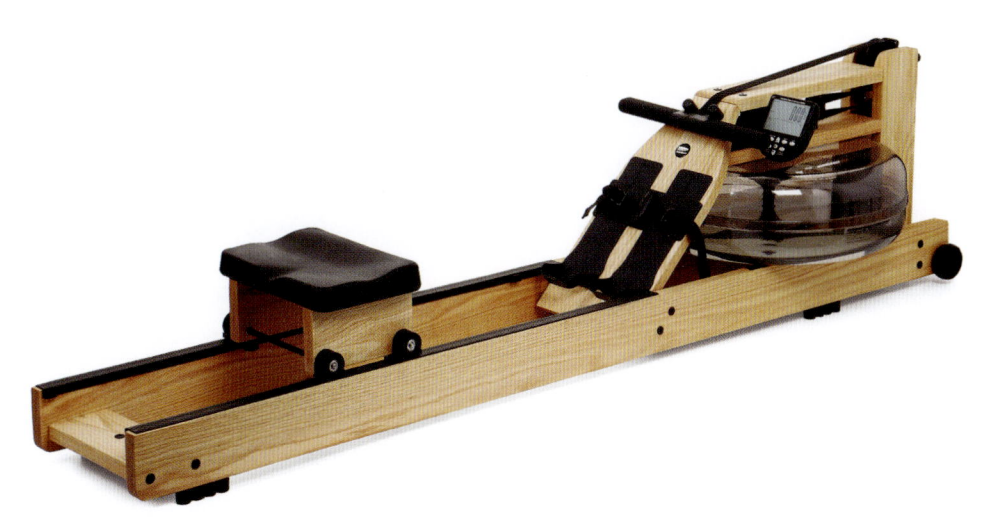

FIGURE 2.2 WaterRower Rowing Machine.
Photo courtesy of WaterRower

resistance through the length of the stroke. To generate intensity or speed, like the air rower, the user must "push" harder off the catch to feel more resistance on the machine.

Water rowers are larger and tend to be more expensive than other rowers. Many people enjoy the sound of the water in the tank as they row. Periodic maintenance is required to maintain the condition of the water in the tank. The water rower is an aesthetically pleasing machine. One drawback is data inconsistency from one machine to the next due to the drag of the stroke depending on the water level in the tank and the water's cleanliness.

Air Rower

Air rowers have historically been the industry standard for the sport of indoor rowing and can be found in boat houses around the world, where they are used for warm-up and training for on-water rowing. Air rowers use a flywheel fan that generates resistance based on the amount of air pulled through the flywheel (see figure 2.3). The more force you push into the foot stretcher, where your feet connect to the machine, the more resistance you'll encounter. This unlimited resistance makes the air rower a great choice for any athlete, from novice to advanced, because the machine will grow with you. As you get stronger and tighten up your technique, you can create the level of resistance you need.

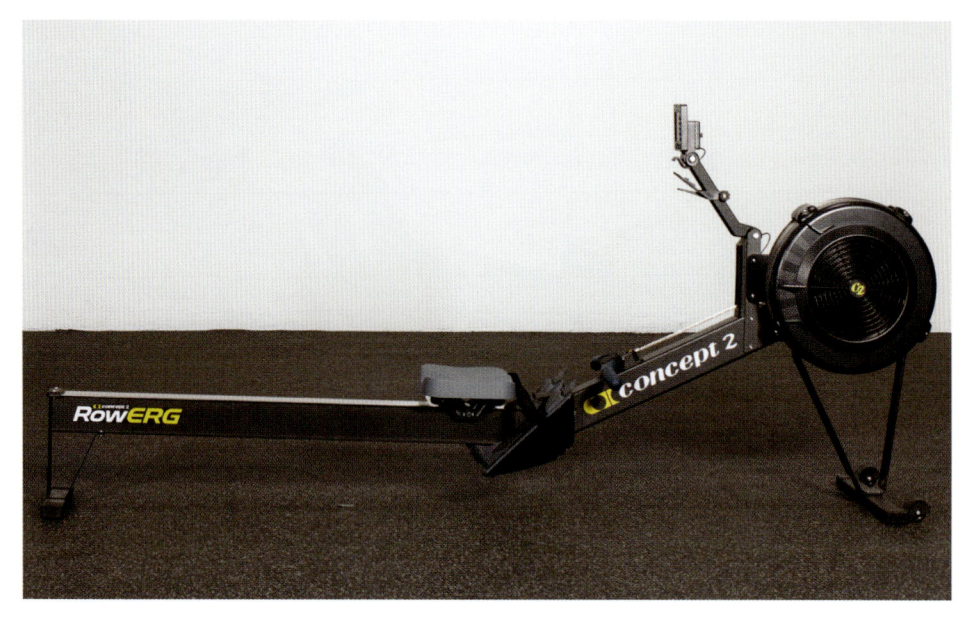

FIGURE 2.3 Concept2 RowErg.

Damper Setting

On an air rower, the damper setting is on the right side of the fan cage. It ranges from 1 to 10 and controls the drag of the flywheel. With the damper set at 10, the fan cage is open, allowing more air to pass across the fan blades, increasing the drag on the flywheel, and making the fan feel heavier. With the damper set at 1, the fan cage is closed, allowing less air to pass across the fan blades, decreasing the drag on the flywheel, and making the fan feel lighter.

Adjusting the damper depends on several factors and isn't as straightforward as "higher is harder." A common misconception about the damper setting is that a higher setting will make the workout more difficult. In fact, the damper is not an accurate unit of resistance measurement, and the damper setting is not universal from one machine to the next. Things like air temperature, machine cleanliness, and even humidity and elevation affect the feeling of the air entering the flywheel. Even the type of workout you do and the type of athlete you are (endurance vs. sprint) will determine how you set the rower to get the most out of it. For example, adjusting the damper a little higher for a short benchmark may allow you to find greater connection to the machine over that shorter time period.

Air rowers offer a smooth stroke that provides a more lifelike feeling of rowing on the water. The data is also more consistent and expansive. Retailing for under $1,000, the popular Concept2 breaks down into smaller parts for easy storage. Maintenance on an air rower includes oiling the chain and wiping down the machine's slide and body. Aside from these things, annual maintenance includes vacuuming the fan.

Magnetic Rower

A series of magnets located close to the flywheel create the resistance on a magnetic rowing machine. The closer the magnets are to the flywheel, the stronger the resistance. Moving the magnets closer or farther away from the flywheel adjusts the resistance. One advantage of a magnetic rowing machine is that it is generally quieter than other types of rowing machines, such as air rowers. They're typically less expensive, take up less room than a water rower, and maintenance is low.

Understanding the type of rowing machine you're using ensures safe and effective usage, enables you to optimize your workouts, facilitates maintenance and repairs, and helps you explore additional features and upgrades available for your machine. When determining which machine to purchase, consider size, price, and how each machine will accommodate your ultimate goals. If you use a rowing machine at a gym or other fitness facility, understand that the type of machine you use can influence its ease of use. If you use more than one type of machine, your performance may vary depending on how the resistance is applied. Rowing is a sport for life, so you'll want to find the machine that works the best for you!

Metrics Used on a Rowing Machine

How do you measure progress on a rower? All rowing machines typically have a built-in display that shows measures of work being done (see figure 2.4). It is important to note that different rowing machines may have variations in their calibration and measurement methods, so the display may not always be directly comparable between different machines. Consult the user's manual if your rower differs from those explained here. Metrics that you'll typically see on your display include distance traveled in meters, wattage, time spent on the rower, 500-meter split time, and calories.

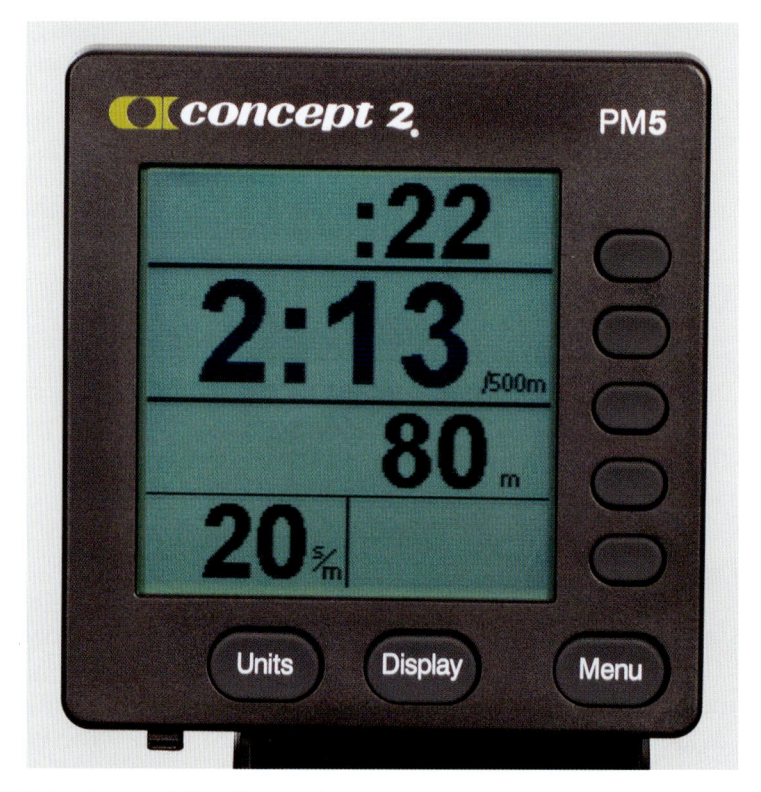

FIGURE 2.4 Concept2 RowErg monitor.

Distance

Distance is the most basic measurement on a rower. Measuring distance on the rowing machine is an important metric for several reasons:

1. *Performance tracking:* Distance measurement allows rowers to track their progress and performance over time. By recording the distance covered during each rowing session, you can see if you are improving or if you need to adjust your training regimen. It provides a tangible and simple measurement of your efforts and helps you set future goals.

2. *Training intensity:* Distance is often used to gauge the intensity of a rowing workout. Rowing machines typically display the time taken to cover a specific distance, allowing you to compare your performance against previous sessions or established benchmarks. You may want to monitor your training intensity and adjust your pace accordingly.

3. *Training programs:* Many rowing training programs and workouts are designed based on specific distances. For example, some programs may prescribe rowing intervals or workouts that involve rowing a certain

distance at varying intensities. Measuring distance ensures that you can accurately follow these programs and achieve the desired training stimulus.

4. *Competition preparation:* Rowers who participate in indoor rowing competitions or use rowing machines as part of their training for outdoor rowing events often need to track their performance in terms of distance. In these scenarios, distance measurement is crucial for assessing competitiveness, setting personal records, and comparing your performance against other athletes.

5. *Motivation and accountability:* Having a distance measurement on the rowing machine can provide motivation and accountability. Seeing progress in terms of the distance covered can be highly motivating, pushing you to surpass your previous achievements. It also allows for friendly competition among rowers, encouraging each person to strive for higher distances and better performances.

Especially if you're new to rowing, distance measurements on a rowing machine help provide basic yet valuable feedback. You may want to track your distance with each workout and take notes about how the workout felt or when you reach a new PR for distance.

> **KEY POINT**
> Distance measurements on a rowing machine help provide basic yet valuable feedback.

Wattage

The wattage on a rower indicates the amount of power generated while rowing. *Power* is defined as the amount of energy consumed per unit of time, or how quickly you perform the work. Work divided by time is the formula to calculate power. On the rower, work happens when you generate force against the foot stretcher. Therefore, power is the level of work you're putting into the machine through the length of the stroke over a certain period. Various factors influence wattage, such as your strength, level of conditioning, and rowing technique. As with all other metrics, the more proficient in rowing you become and the more endurance you build, the higher wattage you should produce over time. Paying attention to the wattage on the rower can be beneficial for several reasons:

1. *Objective measurement:* Wattage provides an objective and quantifiable measurement of your effort and performance. It gives you a clear understanding of the power you are generating, allowing you to track your progress over time and set specific goals for improvement.

2. *Consistency:* Wattage provides a consistent measurement across different types of rowing machines. While factors such as wind resistance or machine calibration can influence metrics like speed and distance, wattage provides a more standardized measurement of your work. This allows for more consistent tracking.

3. *Performance tracking:* Gauging your performance throughout your workout allows you to adjust force (pressure) or stroke rate to maintain a consistent wattage output. This gives you strong parameters for goal setting that allow for adjustment based on specific fitness goals, such as endurance or strength development.

4. *Motivation and accountability:* Wattage provides a common metric for comparison, so if you have a competitive streak, wattage is a great way to compete with others (or yourself)!

> **KEY POINT**
> Work divided by time is the formula to calculate power.

Overall, using wattage on a rowing machine provides a reliable and standardized measurement of your effort. The programs in part IV of the book explain more about how to use wattage as part of your workouts to help you continue to progress and get stronger.

Splits

On the rower, the most common metric used is the 500-meter split. This is an indicator of the time it will take you to row 500 meters in minutes and seconds. Rowing split times can vary greatly based on several factors, including fitness level, technique, and the drag factor or damper setting on the machine (see Damper Setting and Terminology Used in Indoor Rowing for more information on damper setting and drag factor).

The 500-meter split is interchangeable with speed, and it is your rowing speed in the water. Most people who use a rowing machine are concerned with the meters traveled. The lower the split, the more quickly you can cover a set number of meters. There are three ways to get your split lower: pushing harder (generating more force against the foot stretcher), increasing your stroke rate (rowing more strokes over the course of a minute), or both! Using the split on the rower as a training tool can be beneficial for several reasons:

1. *Instant feedback:* Rowing machines automatically calibrate after each stroke and typically display the 500-meter split, or level of intensity, over the last two strokes. This type of feedback allows you to make instant adjustments in your stroke rate or leg pressure (force against the machine) to maintain a specific split time.

2. *Intensity control:* Your rowing workout always depends on the outcome you want to achieve, so it will be based on different intensity levels. The 500-meter split can help you gauge and maintain your desired intensity during a workout.

3. *Consistency:* The 500-meter split is a common and widely recognized metric in the sport of rowing. This allows you to easily compare your performance with others. It is important to note that there will be a difference in split times on different types of rowers. This is based on things like calibration, wind resistance, machine care, or elevation and humidity. Concept2 rowing machines allow for calibration from machine to machine using the drag factor. By identifying the proper drag factor, you can adjust the damper setting to make one machine feel like the next.

4. *Motivation and accountability:* Setting specific split-time goals can provide a clear and targeted goal for your rowing sessions. It's easy to maintain focus when you can bite off pieces of the total distance, knowing that the time it will take you to row the next 500 meters is staring back at you from your monitor. Achieving targeted split times, or PRs (personal records), can be rewarding and keep you motivated to continue to push for the next level.

> **KEY POINT**
>
> The better your form, the lower the split. The lower the split, the more quickly you can cover a set number of meters.

Calories

The rower's calorie display typically shows the estimated number of calories burned during a rowing session. It is based on various factors, such as your body weight, workout intensity, and the duration of the exercise. The rowing machine uses a formula or algorithm to calculate the calories burned based on these inputs. However, it's important to note that the calorie displays on exercise equipment are estimates and may not be entirely accurate for every individual. Why would we use this metric for training?

1. *Variety:* To avoid plateaus and maintain motivation, varying your rowing workouts or how you measure them will keep you engaged.
2. *Training optimization:* Using this as a tool to understand caloric expenditure during different types of training allows you to optimize your training. By tracking calories, you can adjust the duration or intensity of your sessions accordingly. This also helps in comparing rowing to other modalities of exercise, such as running or cycling.

Terminology Used in Indoor Rowing

Some common words used in rowing are defined here. We'll go into more detail about many of these in chapter 3.

- *Catch:* the forward-most part of the stroke and the moment of full compression. When rowing on the water, this is the moment where the blades are behind you and you're setting them into the water to "catch" the resistance of the water.
- *Drive:* the action against the machine that pushes the seat from the front to the back. It is the only part of the stroke where you can generate intensity.
- *Finish:* the backmost part of the stroke. It is the point where your legs are fully extended.
- *Recovery:* the action that returns the seat from the back to the front of the machine.
- *Ratio:* a numerical value that describes the time spent on the drive phase of the stroke compared to the recovery phase of the stroke.
- *Force curve:* a graphical representation of the stroke used to identify areas where you may be breaking the chain of force transfer from the feet to the handle.
- *Drag factor:* a numerical value for the rate at which the flywheel is decelerating. It depends on the workout you're trying to achieve, along with special considerations like experience level, fitness level, or if you're a fast-twitch or slow-twitch athlete.
- *Damper setting:* The adjustable dial on the side of an air rower's fan cage that can be adjusted to control the drag of the flywheel, or how quickly the flywheel slows down. The higher the damper setting the quicker the fan will slow down. The lower the damper setting the longer it will take for the fan to slow.
- *Split time:* The numerical value that is shown as a representation of how long it will take you to row 500 meters at your current stroke rate and pressure.
- *Pace vs. rate: Pace* and *rate* are two terms that many people struggle with; I struggle with them sometimes myself. Rate is just one component that can affect your overall pace, measured in strokes per minute. Pace is "the speed at which you would be moving through the water if you were rowing in a boat. It's expressed as the number of minutes it would take you to row about 500 meters" (Sybertz 2022). In addition to rate, power also plays a role in your overall pace.

3. *Motivation and accountability:* Seeing the number of calories burned over time may offer a sense of accomplishment and keep you motivated to work harder to increase that number.

The actual number of calories burned can vary depending on an individual's metabolism and other factors. For this reason, it's important to use this metric as more of an estimate than an exact measure when working through your training.

Understanding each of the metrics on the rower display allows you to incorporate them into setting specific fitness goals, tracking your progress in different ways, and optimizing your training plan for better results.

Rowing has a highly technical aspect, and understanding the specific lingo allows you to grasp and implement the nuances of proper rowing technique. It also allows you to get the most out of your machine and your stroke! Now that you know the lingo, let's get into how to row properly and efficiently in chapter 3.

PART II

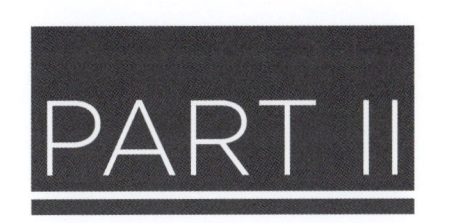

LEARN PROPER ROWING

3

ROWING TECHNIQUE

As you learned in part I, rowing is a low-impact exercise that engages multiple muscle groups and provides an excellent cardiorespiratory workout. Proper technique is essential to maximizing the benefits of indoor rowing while minimizing the risk of injury. You also learned that rowing activates all of the major muscle groups in your body as well as a majority of the supporting muscles—but did you know that to access that level of activation, you must row well? It is helpful to understand how your body works with the rowing machine. We'll look at three contributing factors here that will help you get the most out of your rowing workouts: drag factor, foot stretcher setup, and stroke sequence.

Drag Factor

One of the most common misconceptions in rowing is that the damper setting sets the machine's resistance. In fact, the damper simply controls the fan's drag, or how quickly the fan will slow down. Pushing harder away from the front of the machine is the only way that you'll grab greater resistance on the rower. Drag factor is a numerical value for the rate at which the blade or the flywheel decelerates, or how fast the fan slows down after each push. Air rowers have a monitor setting that allows you to adjust the damper setting (explained in chapter 2) to calibrate the machine so that one machine is consistent with the next. Determining the drag factor on an indoor rower is a key aspect of optimizing your rowing experience. The drag factor is essentially a measure of the resistance you feel when pulling the handle during a rowing stroke.

> **KEY POINT**
>
> Determining the drag factor on an indoor rower is a key aspect of optimizing your rowing experience.

All things considered, you're looking for a drag factor that allows you to find the most connection with the machine from your feet to your fingertips. When connection happens, it's a magical moment when all the muscles fire and there are no breaks in the chain of connection between the feet and the fingertips. While a general range for drag factor is from 100 to 125, it depends on the workout you're trying to achieve, along with special considerations like experience level or if you're a fast-twitch or slow-twitch athlete.

Special Considerations for Drag Factor

Special considerations for drag factor preference include experience level and fast-twitch or slow-twitch muscle fiber concentration. Understanding the type of athlete you are and how your body works with the machine will allow you to get more out of each stroke. Let's start with experience level.

Experience Level

As you become more masterful with the biomechanics of the rowing stroke, you make a better connection with the machine based on the timing of your stroke. This simply means that your muscles fire when they should, in the order that makes the most impact. You're able to understand how quickly to push away from the front of the machine to make the biggest impact, and you don't need the flywheel to keep resistance on the chain for you.

Slow-Twitch Athlete Versus Fast-Twitch Athlete

Athletes who have developed a higher concentration of slow-twitch muscle fibers (endurance athletes, marathon runners) might lack the explosiveness out of the catch needed to catch the spinning flywheel at lower settings. These athletes might better transfer the force of the leg drive into the handle at a higher damper setting.

Contrary to that, more explosive athletes (sprinters, Crossfit athletes) have developed a higher concentration of fast-twitch muscle fibers and can put a good bit of force into the machine at the turnaround from the recovery through the catch into the drive. These athletes might better transfer the force of the leg drive into the handle at a lower damper setting.

On the Concept2 rower, for example, you can set your drag factor by changing the damper setting, using the monitor to calibrate the machine. Press Menu on the performance monitor and select More Options and Display Drag Factor. From there, you'll row a few strokes, and the drag factor will display (figure 3.1). Per the Concept2 website (n.d.), "a brand new RowErg will have a drag factor of 90 or less at a damper setting of 1 and 200 or more at a damper setting of 10. These drag factor ranges for new ergs assumes that the machines are at sea level."

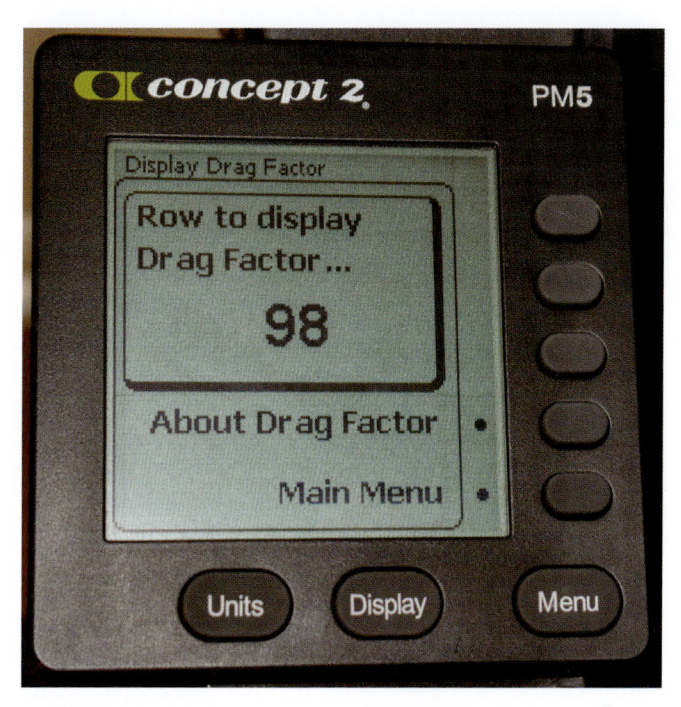

FIGURE 3.1 Performance monitor 5 drag factor display.

Foot Stretcher Setup

The first step in proper rowing technique is proper erg setup, starting with the foot stretcher. This is important because it will allow you to get into a strong catch position. That strong catch is the origin of the leg drive, or the moment when the rower applies the most force. By adjusting the foot stretcher height, you adjust the hip angle as you come into the catch. If it's too high, you won't be able to bring your body all the way forward into the catch and use the legs completely. If it's too low, you may overcompress at the catch position, losing the connection in the core that you need to drive away quickly.

To set up your foot stretcher, adjust the pegboard so the strap runs across the widest part of the foot or the top shoelace (see figure 3.2). Make sure that the strap is tight across the foot. Note that you can adjust this later to best suit your body and any possible restrictions or modifications.

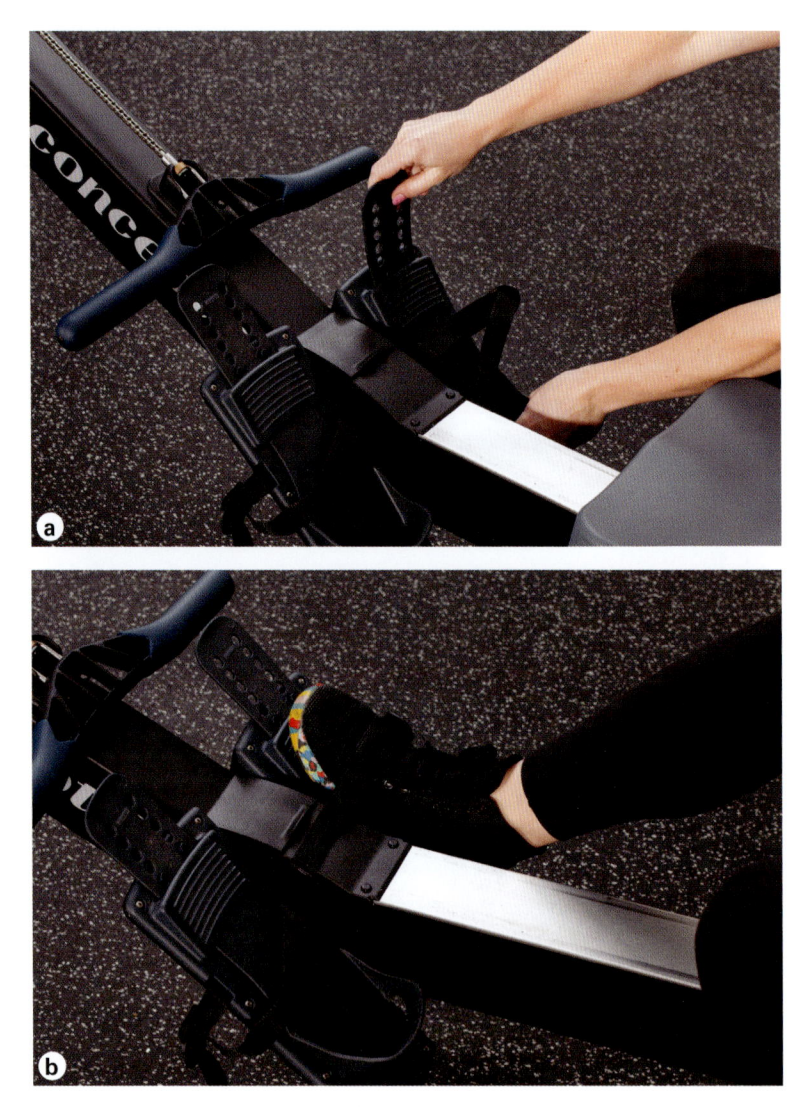

FIGURE 3.2 Set up the foot stretcher by adjusting the pegboard to the proper location, with the strap running across the widest part of the foot.

The rower is so versatile that it accommodates most restrictions or limitations. Possible restrictions include tight hamstrings, a tight lower back, lack of mobility in the ankles or hips, pregnancy, or being overweight. Lowering the heel closer to the floor can accommodate these restrictions by lessening the angle from the hips to the knees and allowing more space for your body to move forward. The rule of thumb is to not go so low that the strap inhibits your toes' movement.

Once you have set the drag factor and foot stretcher, it's time to dial in your technique! Let's dive a little further into the four parts of the stroke sequence: the catch, the drive, the finish, and the recovery. Tightening up your technique in all parts of the stroke will engage the most muscles and allow for the highest reward.

> **KEY POINT**
>
> The rower is so versatile that it accommodates most restrictions or limitations.

Stroke Sequence

To maximize power and efficiency on the rower, the stroke should always follow the sequence of legs, body, arms on the drive, and arms, body, legs on the recovery. We'll break down each phase of the stroke here: the catch, the drive, the finish, and the recovery.

> **KEY POINT**
>
> To maximize power and efficiency on the rower, the stroke should always follow the sequence of legs, body, arms on the drive, and arms, body, legs on the recovery.

The Catch

In indoor rowing, the term *catch position* refers to the initial position of the rowing stroke; on the water, this is where the rower's oar or paddle enters the water. Achieving a proper catch position, as shown in figure 3.3, is crucial for an effective and efficient rowing stroke. Here are some key points about the catch position in indoor rowing.

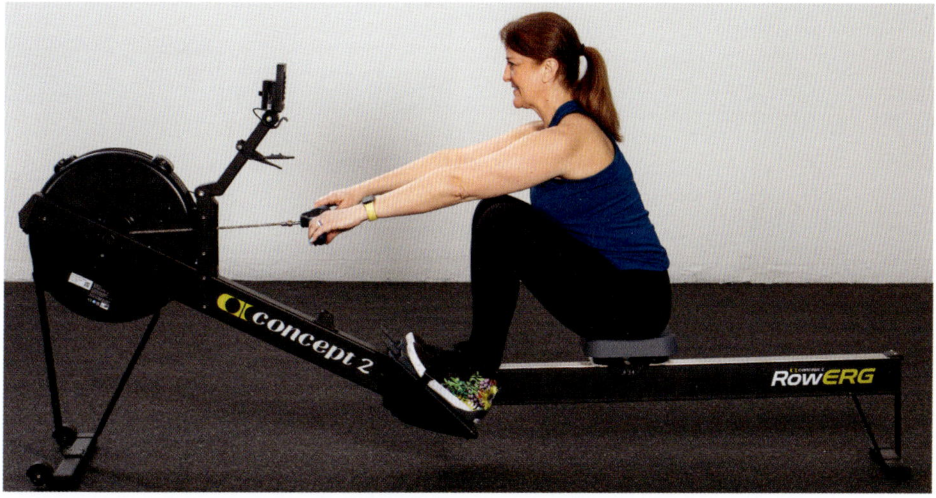

FIGURE 3.3 The catch position of the stroke.

Body Position
- Sit at the front of the rowing machine with your knees bent and your shins vertical, with your knees above your ankles. Strap your feet securely into the footrests. A slight heel lift is okay if it is natural, not forced.
- Activate your latissimus dorsi, serratus anterior, pectoralis major and minor, and lower trapezius muscles to depress the scapula and brace the core.
- Hinge your body forward so that your shoulders are in front of your hips. If there were a clock on your right wall, your shoulders would be at 11 o'clock and your hips at four o'clock.
- Avoid rounding through the spine or tucking the tailbone because poor posture can cause pain in the lower back.

Arms and Shoulders
- Fully extend your arms in front of you, reaching toward the flywheel or resistance mechanism.
- Relax and slightly protract (press forward) your shoulders. They should not shrug or be pressed down.
- Avoid overreaching with your upper body because this can cause pain in the lower back.

Force Curve

The force curve is a graphical representation of the stroke. It's an important tool because it provides information on the continuity of your stroke (or how much time you keep the handle under tension) and how it affects power output. By analyzing the force curve, you can identify areas where you may be breaking the chain of force transfer from the feet to the handle. An ideal force curve should be smooth and symmetrical, with one peak in the middle (see figure 3.4). Any variances in the force curve will give you a road map of pieces of the stroke or areas of your technique that might need attention. The monitor analyzes the force curve based on the level of resistance maintained on the chain over time.

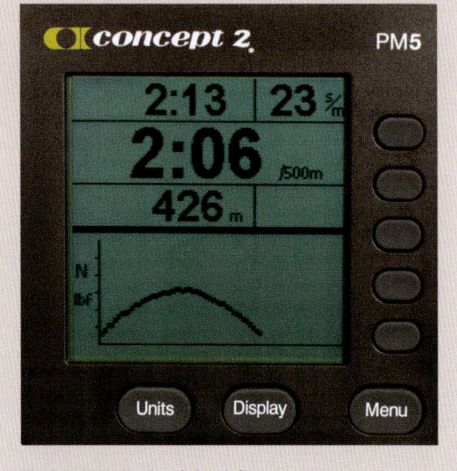

FIGURE 3.4 Ideal force curve.

Hands and Grip
- Hold the handle in a relaxed, overhand grip, slightly wider than shoulder-width, depending on your comfort and the specific rowing machine design.
- Keep your wrists flat.
- Avoid gripping too tightly because this can cause undue stress on the forearms and hands and waste energy.

Finding a strong catch will allow you to set your body to efficiently transfer force from your legs to the handle, maximizing the benefits of each stroke while minimizing the risk of injury. Regular practice and attention to form can help you refine your catch position and improve your overall indoor rowing performance.

The Drive

The drive phase of the stroke shown in figure 3.5 is the work phase. This is the only part of the stroke where you can generate power, so it is critical to ensure that you're following the proper sequence of legs, body, arms throughout the drive. The leg muscles are the largest and strongest muscle group in the body, contributing about 60% of the work during the rowing stroke. Once the knees extend, the upper body maintains the acceleration the lower body initiated, performing an additional 30% of the work as the body swings open. From here, the arms finish the last 10% as they move quickly into the chest and then back out to initiate the recovery phase.

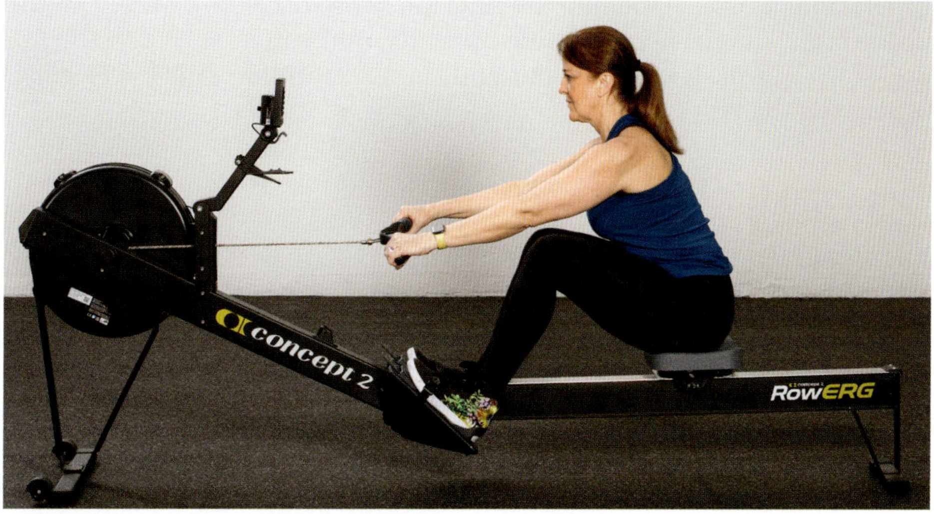

FIGURE 3.5 The drive phase of the stroke.

KEY POINT

The drive is the only part of the stroke where you can generate power, so it is critical to ensure that you're following the proper sequence of legs, body, arms throughout the drive.

Body Position
- Brace your core.
- Keep your shoulders in front of your hips throughout the drive until you almost fully extend your knees.
- After extending your knees, swing your body back and pull the handle to your sternum.

Arms and Shoulders
- Extend your arms fully through the drive to the finish.

Hands and Grip
- Once your body swings open, pull the handle to your chest.

Moving out of the catch position, the lower abdominal muscles brace to protect the lower back, and the hamstrings contract to initiate the force against the foot stretcher. The quadriceps femoris muscle group (rectus femoris, vastus lateralis, vastus medialis, and vastus intermedius) extends the knees. As the knees extend, the back muscles (latissimus dorsi, lower and upper trapezius, rhomboids, and erector spinae) work in conjunction with the gluteus muscles to swing the hips open. The biceps and deltoids will activate to finish the stroke by pulling the handle to the chest.

One of the most common stroke errors—opening the hips too soon or leading with the shoulders—happens on the drive, causing a less efficient generation of force. Opening the hips too soon forces you to rely on the upper body and back to generate intensity, and you miss out on the full use of leg power. It can also put additional strain on your lower back, increasing the risk of injury.

The Finish

The finish is essentially the transfer from the drive into the recovery phase. The finish is an active position at the back of the rowing stroke. The legs fully extend through the ankles, knees, and hips; the torso leans back; and the handle pulls into the chest, as shown in figure 3.6.

Body Position
- Sit at the back of the rowing machine with your knees, ankles, and hips extended. Press your feet down against the foot stretcher. Keeping your entire foot pressed down is important.

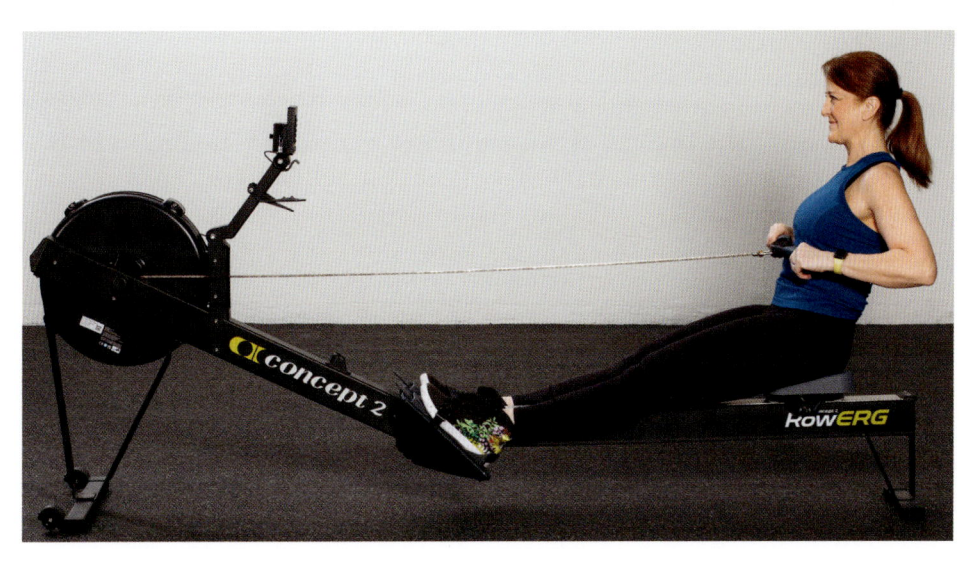

FIGURE 3.6 The finish position of the stroke.

- Hinge your body back so that your shoulders are behind your hips. If there were a clock on your right wall, your shoulders would now be at one o'clock and your hips at seven o'clock.
- Activate the back extensors and the abdominals to keep your torso engaged as you hinge back.

Arms and Shoulders
- Engage the biceps, deltoids, latissimus dorsi, and wrist extensors to hold the handle at your chest.
- Relax and slightly depress your shoulders.
- Pull your elbows back and down at 45 degrees; and keep your wrists flat.
- Avoid excessively leaning back, because this does not add any value on an indoor rower and can cause pain in the lower back.

Hands and Grip
- Hands should be relaxed and holding the handle in the finger tips.
- Wrists should be flat and not flexed.

The finish of the stroke should always be considered a "pass-through" phase. Although your legs stay extended and hold for a moment, the arms will tap away from the chest, keeping your body moving right into the recovery phase.

The Recovery

The recovery phase of the rowing stroke (see figure 3.7) happens as you move from the back of the machine to the front. The recovery is a great chance to catch your breath, collect yourself, and set up your next powerful drive.

Body Position
- Hinge your body forward from the hips to get the handle across the knees before they bend.
- Keep your legs extended until the handle passes your knees.
- Keep your entire foot, including the toes, connected to the foot stretcher.
- Once your knees bend, move two to three times slower than you did on the drive.

Arms and Shoulders
- Move your arms away first.
- Transition your shoulders from behind the hips (one o'clock) to in front of the hips (11 o'clock).

Hands and Grip
- Cradle the handle in your fingertips.

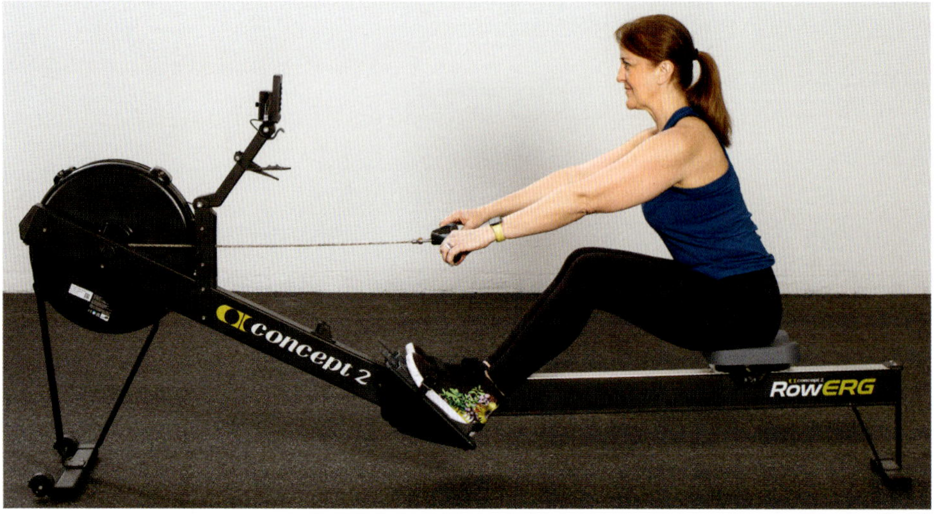

FIGURE 3.7 The recovery phase of the stroke.

From the finish position, smoothly send the hands away from your body. Next, the body swings forward, allowing the stroke to stay in motion. Then, after the handle has passed over the knees, and the body has arrived at the 11 o'clock position, the knees bend. You'll want to think of this as a controlled return to the front of the machine. The more control you have through your recovery, the more powerful you can be as you transition through the catch.

It is important to note that the sequence of the recovery is arms, body, legs, and the ratio of the stroke on the recovery will always be two to three times slower than it is on the drive.

Ratio

In rowing, the term *ratio* refers to the relationship between the time spent on the drive phase and the recovery phase of the stroke. When rowing indoors, you apply force to the foot stretcher during the drive phase to generate power. The recovery phase of the stroke is when you're relaxing back to the catch position to set up for the next strong drive.

Ratio is a numerical value that is important for achieving an efficient stroke. The drive will always be quicker than the recovery. A 2:1 ratio means that you spend twice as much time on the recovery phase as you do on the drive phase. This is necessary so that the flywheel has time to spin and allow meters to tick up. A rushed recovery or lack of quickness on the drive is an indicator of an inefficient stroke, which will compromise the level of power or speed you may achieve. The machine does not measure the ratio; it changes as your stroke rate goes up or down. The lower the stroke rate, the bigger the difference in your timing (i.e., pushing back quickly and returning to the front very slowly would be a 3:1 ratio). The higher the stroke rate, the smaller the difference in your timing (i.e., pushing back quickly and coming back slowly would be a 2:1 ratio).

Key points to remember when rowing:
- Body sequencing is imperative on the drive (legs, body, arms) and recovery (arms, body, legs) to access the highest amount of muscle and provide the strongest connection to the rowing machine. When you connect with the machine, you take the force that you generate and allow it to move from your feet through your body to your handles. Any breaks in your connection (bent elbows, overcompressed knees, rounded spine, early hip opening), will dampen the force from your legs before it gets to the handle to make the flywheel move.

- Smooth, continuous motion is crucial for efficient rowing. Avoid pausing at the finish.
- Focus on leg drive to generate power rather than pulling with your arms.
- Keep in mind that the drive is always quicker than the recovery.

Keep practicing! In rowing, practice makes progress. Continually review or have someone else review your stroke. Rowing will provide you with countless results when done properly.

4

COMMON ERRORS IN ROWING

As we described in chapter 3, the goal when using the rower is connection from the feet to the fingertips! Typically, anything that compromises the connection to the machine will drain power from the stroke. We now know that the rowing sequence is critical and foundational in finding power on the drive. Using the legs to initiate the stroke, following through with the body, and then the arms allows us to use the large leg muscles to do the bulk of the work.

There are several common errors that people can make when using the erg. The most critical ones cause a loss of power and break the chain from the feet to the fingers. Let's look at some common errors and how to correct them with drills that help you practice each phase of the stroke sequence.

Bending the Knees Too Soon

The recovery sequence of the rowing stroke is likely the most difficult portion of the stroke for new rowers. The recovery is the part of the stroke that takes us from the back to the front of the machine. Each recovery phase should first extend the arms, then swing or hinge the body forward, and finally bend the knees. Bending your knees too soon on the recovery—before your hands have passed over your knees on the way forward (see figure 4.1)—can cause you to lose the power and momentum generated during the drive phase of the stroke, as well as disrupt the fluidity of the rowing motion.

To execute a proper recovery in rowing, wait until your hands have passed over your knees and your body is over your thighs before you begin to bend them. This allows you to set your hips in a closed position, thus loading the hamstrings and glutei (glutes) to work hard on the drive.

The best drills to do to correct this error are the body over pause drill and the double pause drill.

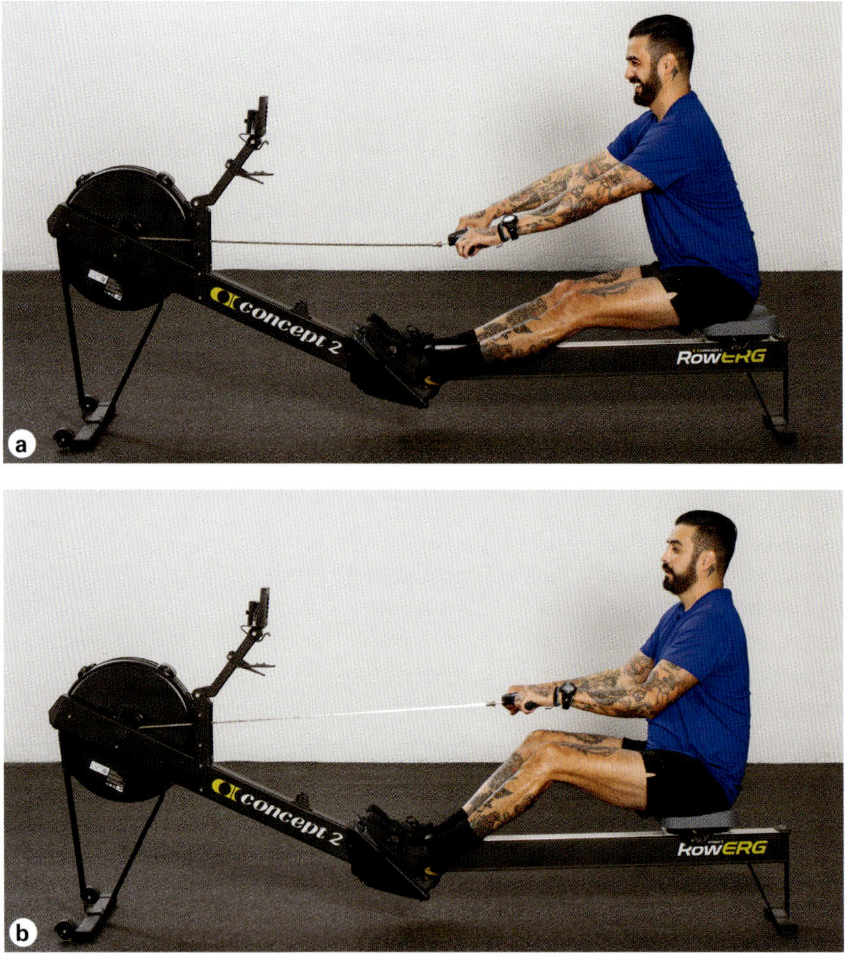

FIGURE 4.1 *(a)* Proper versus *(b)* improper form through the recovery phase of the rowing sequence.

KEY POINT
To execute a proper recovery in rowing, wait until your hands have passed over your knees before you begin to bend them.

BODY OVER PAUSE AND DOUBLE PAUSE DRILLS

These drills will usually fix a host of stroke errors, including rushing the recovery and lacking a hip hinge. Posture and a good hip hinge are important.

- Start in a strong catch position with good posture *(a)*, with the shoulders in front of the hips and arms reaching forward. Engage the latissimus dorsi (lats) and brace the belly.
- Push back through the drive and, keeping the legs down, send the arms and body forward into the *body over* position, meaning that the handle has passed the knees and the torso is forward to the 11 o'clock position with the hips behind the shoulders. Remember that hinging from the hips is critical *(b)*. Pause for three counts.

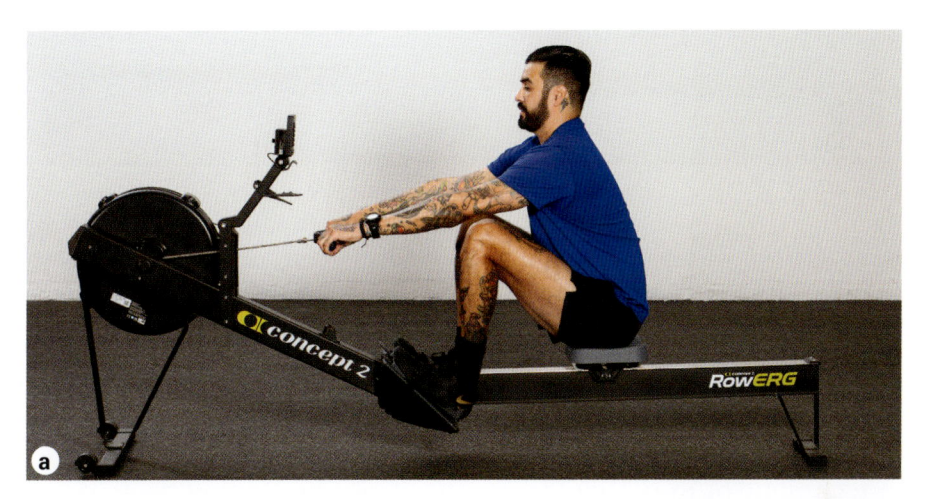

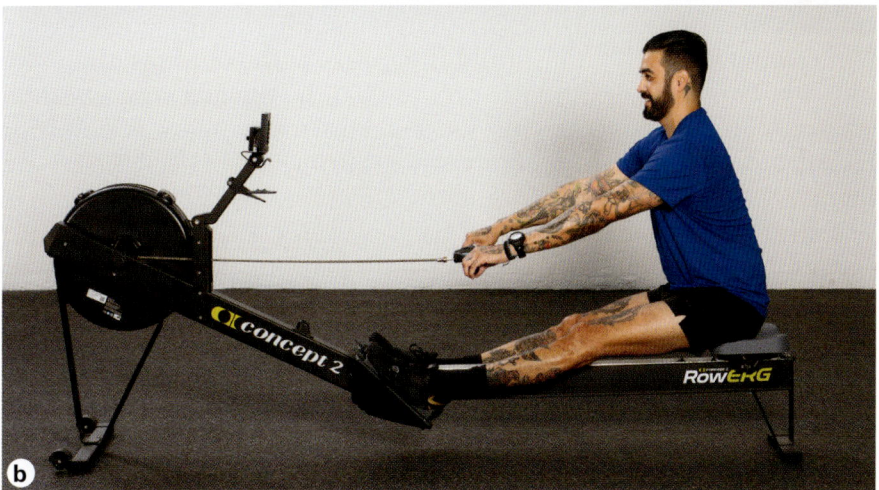

(continued)

Body Over Pause and Double Pause drills *(continued)*

- Move through the recovery sequence slowly, right through the catch into the next quick drive *(c)*.

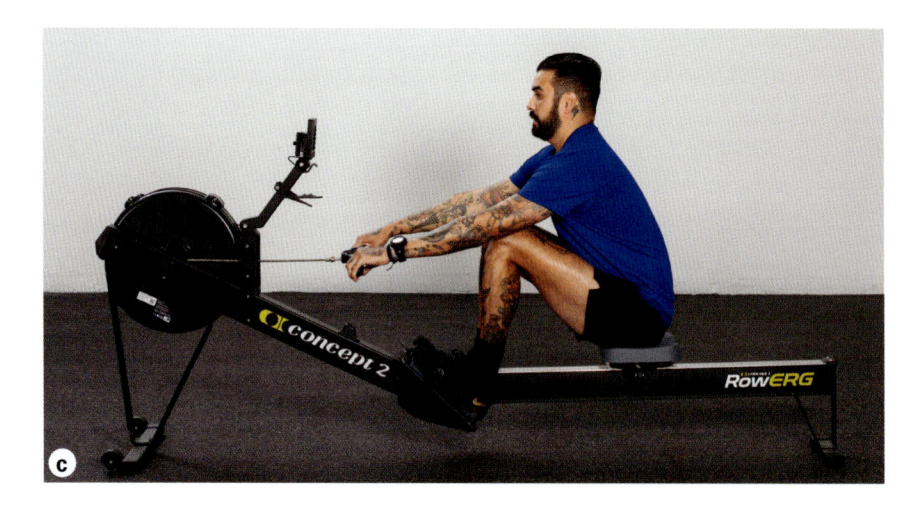

To make this a double pause drill, add a three-count pause after the arms release forward from the finish position and then again once the torso swings forward to close the hips.

Leading With the Body

On the rowing machine, *leading with the shoulders* refers to the incorrect technique of initiating the rowing stroke by leaning back with the shoulders first (figure 4.2), rather than engaging the legs and core first. When rowing properly, you should first press with your legs, then swing back with your core, and finally pull the handle toward your chest with your arms and shoulders. This sequence of movements is commonly referred to as the *leg drive, body swing, arm pull* or *legs, body, arms* sequence. Leading with the shoulders can create inefficient rowing and cause strain on the shoulders and back muscles. It can also put a large amount of pressure on the hip flexor muscles, causing chronic hip pain and tightness.

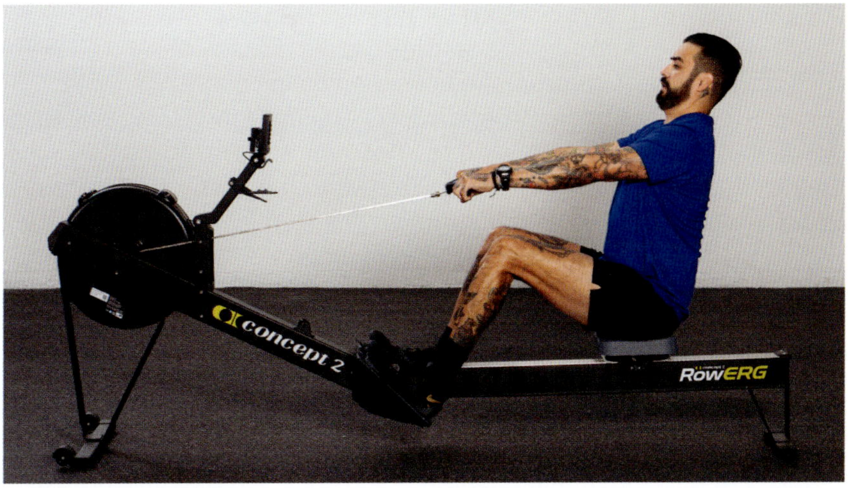

FIGURE 4.2 Incorrect form during the drive phase by leading with the shoulders and having them behind the hips.

To execute a proper drive in rowing, maintain a forward hinged position as you're extending through your knees. This forward hinge allows you to engage the hamstrings and glutes to initiate the drive. A good way to practice this technique is to start each stroke by pushing off with your legs and focusing on the feeling of power coming from your lower body rather than your upper body.

> **KEY POINT**
> To execute a proper drive in rowing, maintain a forward hinged position as you're extending through your knees.

The best drill to fix this error is the legs only pick drill.

LEGS ONLY PICK DRILL

This drill can be used anytime you're not experiencing core engagement on the drive, causing a lack of power from the legs. The drill starts with only the legs, continues the stroke sequence, and finishes with a full stroke. Make sure that your abdominal muscles tighten as you return to the catch position to protect your back on the next drive. Throughout the drill, continue to reinforce the connection from the feet to the handles.

- Start in a strong catch position with good posture, with the shoulders in front of the hips at 11 o'clock and arms reaching forward. Engage the lats and brace the belly *(a)*.
- *Legs only:* Keep the arms and body forward and drive back with only the legs *(b)*. Do not change the position of the arms and upper body. Keep the core tight and engaged through the drive and the recovery; maintain the proper 2:1 ratio of drive to recovery; and note that your body should hang from the handle.

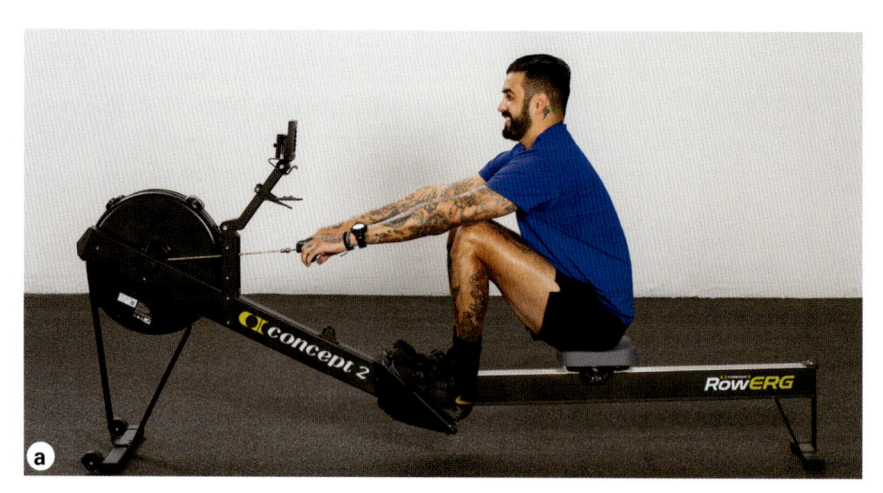

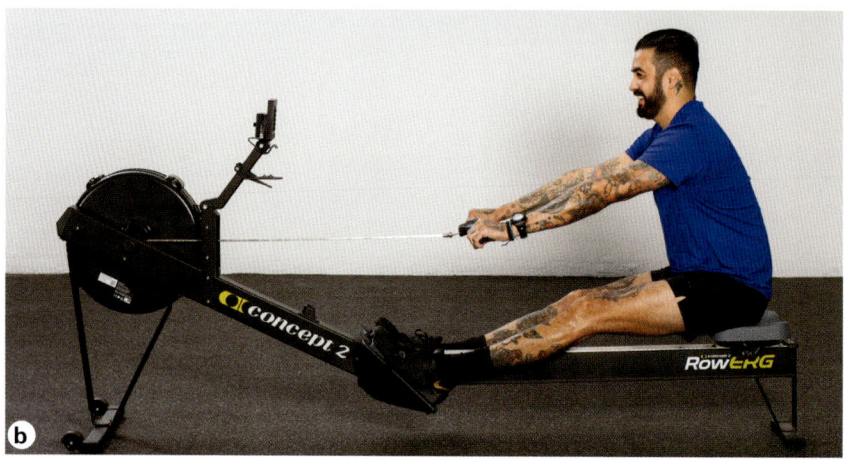

- *Legs and body:* Once you start to find power with the legs only, add in the body, opening the hips and the torso to one o'clock *(c)*.
- *Legs, body, arms:* Once the legs and body (90% of the stroke) are solid, add in the arms. Maintain the stroke ratio throughout the entire drill: quick drive and slower recovery *(d)*.

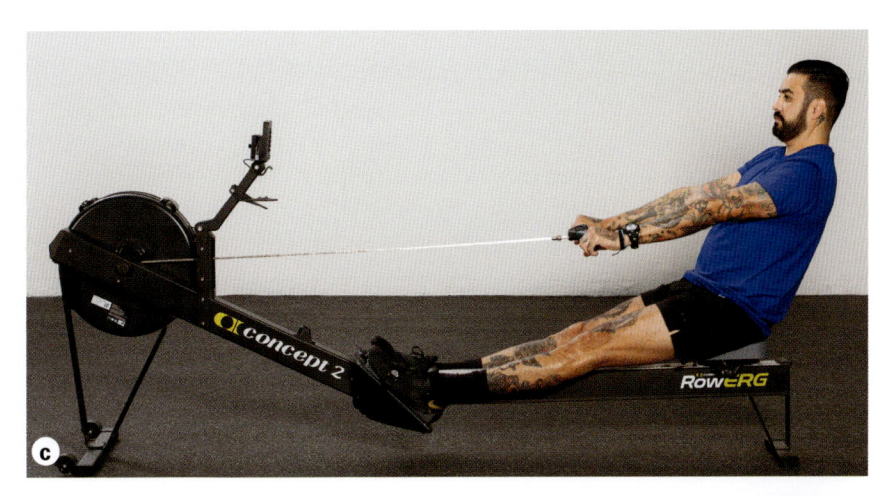

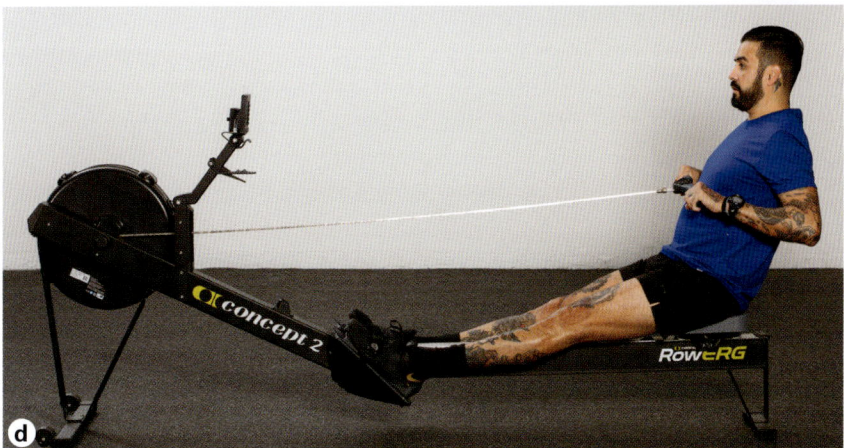

Common Misconceptions About Rowing

There are a lot of misconceptions about rowing. Here we discuss the most prominent misconceptions and briefly explain why they are, in fact, misconceptions. It's important to understand what rowing is and is not, and why it's such a great exercise option.

Misconception 1: Rowing is mainly an arm workout.

Rowing is a full-body exercise that engages multiple muscle groups and is mostly a leg-driven sport! During the stroke, your legs drive first, taking the brunt of the work. As you extend through your legs, your core muscles stabilize your body and help maintain proper posture. This transfers the force from the legs to the arms, and the arms finish the stroke. Using the larger muscles of the legs not only allows you to access more power on each stroke but also allows you to expend more energy and burn more calories. While rowing primarily targets your legs and core, you also get a great arm workout. Just remember that the stroke is 60% legs, 30% core, and only 10% arms!

Misconception 2: Indoor rowing is too hard or too easy.

Whether rowing is considered too hard or too easy depends on various factors, including an individual's fitness level, technique, and experience. When done with proper technique, rowing can be a demanding cardiorespiratory exercise that engages multiple muscle groups. To get the most out of the workout, you must understand ratio and timing, as well as have a heightened level of body awareness to engage the right muscles at the right time.

The beauty of the rowing machine is that it is effort based. To make it hard, you must push hard! To make it easier, just push a little less. This makes it a great modality for all fitness levels. As you get stronger and more in tune with your technique, the machine and your workout grow with you, allowing you to increase your level of challenge.

Misconception 3: To go further, I must row faster.

In rowing, stroke rate refers to the number of strokes or rowing movements you take per minute. While stroke rate is an important factor in rowing, simply increasing your stroke rate alone may not necessarily make you go faster. There are several factors to consider when optimizing your rowing speed and efficiency. Finding a connection to the machine allows for the most efficient use of the machine to "go further" on each stroke.

Stroke rate, how quickly you move up and down the slide, affects the rhythm and pace of your rowing, and finding the right balance is crucial. A higher stroke rate generally allows you to take more strokes per minute, which may result in a lower split and more meters. However, if you increase your stroke rate without maintaining proper technique and power, it may lead to a less effective stroke and decreased efficiency.

Misconception 4: Rowing is bad for my back.

Concerns about rowing causing back injuries are common. However, when performed with proper technique and form, rowing is a low-impact exercise that can strengthen the back and improve posture. It is important to maintain good posture and engage the core muscles to support the back during the rowing motion. Immobility in the hips or inflexible hamstrings or glutes can cause lower back pain. Rowing takes your body through a full range of motion, from triple flexion to triple extension, working your hip mobility and stretching and strengthening your hamstrings and glutes with each stroke.

Misconception 5: A high damper setting will give you the best workout.

People often confuse damper setting with resistance or intensity. The damper setting is not a unit of measurement. It's merely a control that will let more or less air into the flywheel. The only true measure of intensity is the drag factor, which uses the deceleration of the fan to determine how much work the rower is doing.

When completing a workout, it's best to choose the drag factor that is suited for the goal of the workout. Longer distances might choose a lower drag factor (or a lower damper setting), while shorter sprint distances might adjust to a higher drag. It's important to know that the best rowers in the world don't row with their damper set at 10. It's all about learning how to generate the intensity yourself, not relying on the machine to do it for you; that's when the real work happens!

It is important to dispel misconceptions because they stand in the way of learning something new! Although the sport of rowing has been around for decades, rowing as a fitness modality is new and fresh. It's time to move beyond what we think we know into a place of growth!

Early Arm Pull

This error occurs when you initiate the movement with your arms instead of your legs and core (figure 4.3), resulting in a weaker stroke and diminished power. Originating the stroke from the arms does not fully engage the muscles in your legs, core, and back that are crucial for generating power and maintaining proper form. Pulling with the arms too soon may also increase the risk of injury by putting unnecessary strain on the shoulders and arms.

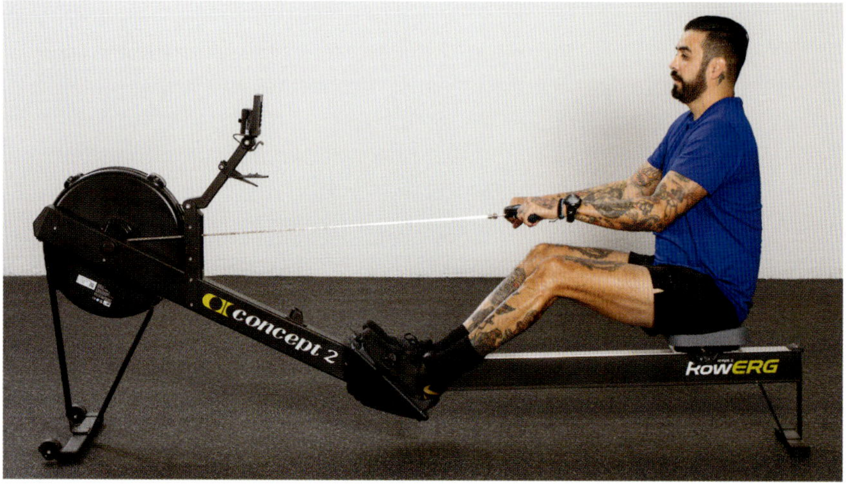

FIGURE 4.3 Incorrect form during the drive phase by initiating the movement with the arms instead of your legs and core.

To avoid pulling with your arms too soon, focus on driving through your legs first and then following through with your body and arms. It's important to remember that the arms are just one part of the rowing stroke and that the power should come primarily from your legs and core. Once your legs fully extend, start your hinge back to the finish position, opening your hips and engaging your core. Pull the handle toward your sternum with your arms for the final phase of the drive. Begin the movement by pushing down and away with your feet, keeping your arms straight and your core engaged. Think of your arms as steel cables that connect your body to the handle; they are strong and unyielding, but limber. By using proper technique and focusing on engaging the right muscles at the right time, you can improve your rowing performance and reduce the risk of injury.

KEY POINT

To avoid pulling with your arms too soon, focus on driving through your legs first and then following through with your body and arms.

The best drill to help fix this error is the heavy handle drill.

HEAVY HANDLE DRILL

For this drill, you will need a partner or resistance band. While seated on the rower, have your partner kneel next to the flywheel of your machine.

- Take the handle in your hands, fully extend your arms, and sit in the catch position. Your partner should also grab the handle with both hands *(a)*.
- When you're ready, you'll both pull the handle in opposite directions, creating resistance on the handle. Leverage the press against the foot stretcher to feel your core activate. You can only do this with extended arms.
- If you don't have a partner to assist you, wrap a heavy resistance band around your handle and your flywheel *(b)*. As you press away, let the band pull your arms straight.

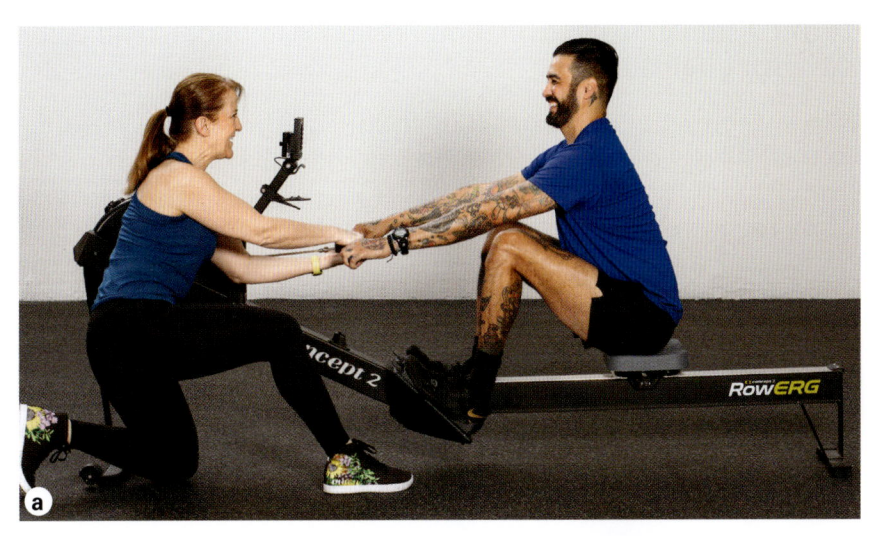

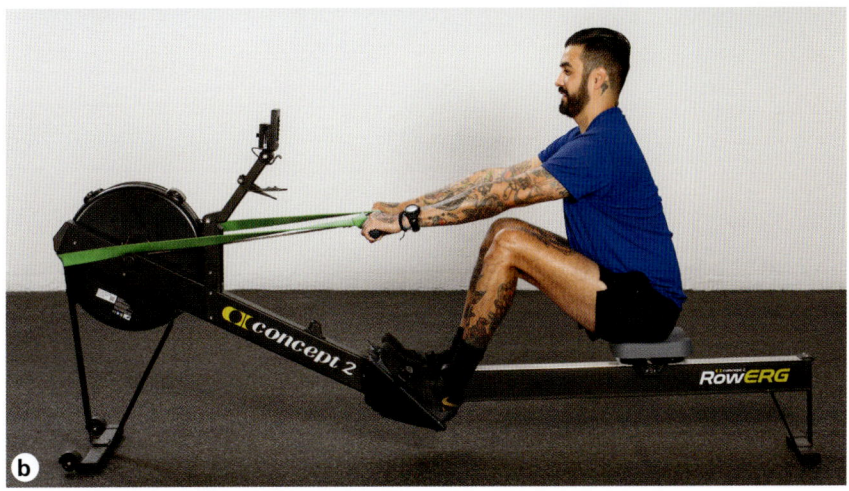

Overcompression

Overcompression happens at the catch when the knees pass beyond the ankles and the shins pass beyond vertical (figure 4.4). This error can happen for several reasons, including lacking a hip hinge in the recovery, rushing the recovery, pulling the foot straps through the recovery, and setting the foot stretcher too low. Address this error quickly because overcompression can cause hyperflexion in the knees, which can ultimately cause chronic knee pain or ligament damage from direct sheer and compressive force on the posterior tibia.

The first step in fixing overcompression is to understand where the error originates. It could be a simple fix of keeping the heels down or raising the positioning on the foot stretcher. Once you determine the issue, this will help you identify how to fix it.

> **KEY POINT**
>
> The first step in fixing overcompression is to understand where the error originates.

To fix overcompression caused by lacking a hip hinge or rushing the recovery, the body over pause drill on page 43 will help. To fix overcompression caused by rushing the recovery or pulling the foot straps, the strapless rowing drill on page 53 will help. You can also place a towel on your slide about six inches (15 cm) from the front of the slide to give a tactile cue that you're close enough to the catch.

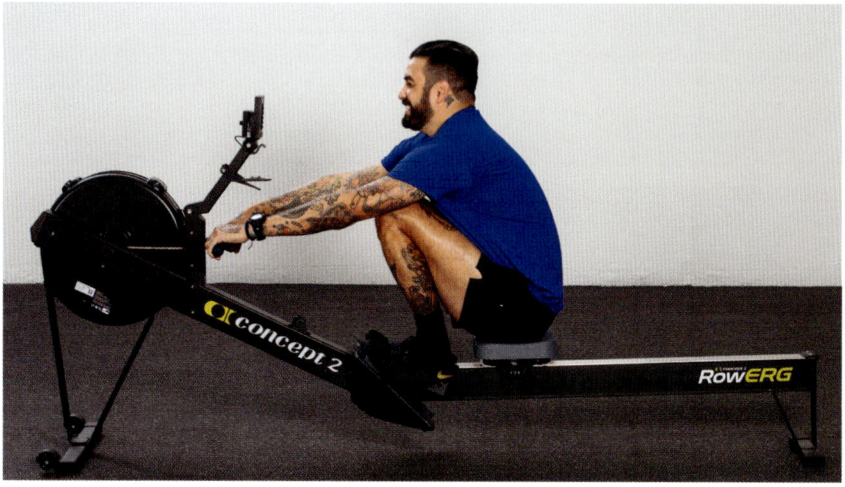

FIGURE 4.4 Overcompression at the catch.

STRAPLESS ROWING DRILL

The purpose of the strapless rowing drill is to reinforce connection to the rower through core engagement and always keeping the entire foot in contact with the foot stretcher when rowing. This drill can fix a lack of core engagement at the finish (using the straps to hold the one o'clock position), rushing the recovery (using the straps to pull yourself back to the catch position), and excessive layback (leaning beyond one o'clock at the finish).

- Start in a strong catch position with good posture, with the shoulders in front of the hips and arms reaching forward. Engage the lats and brace the belly. Note that the feet should be *on top* of the straps *(a)*.
- Push away gently on the first drive, remembering that you don't have the straps to hold your feet to the foot stretcher.
- Push back into a full stroke, maintaining a complete connection between the foot stretcher and the foot (from the balls of the feet to the heels) *(b)*.
- As you continue rowing, keep building pressure through the legs, focusing on engagement through the core to increase the intensity and lower the split.

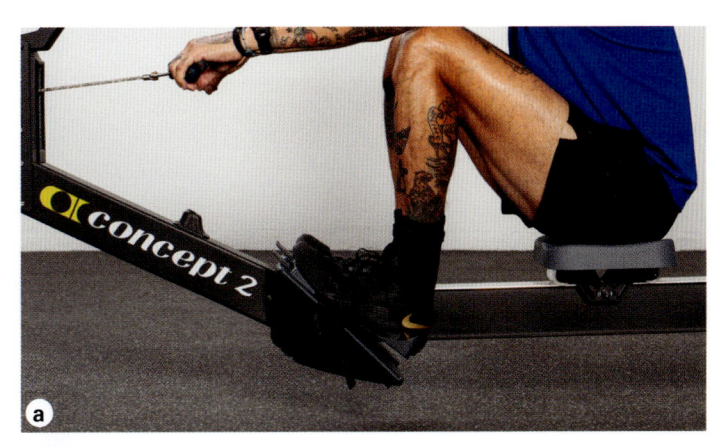

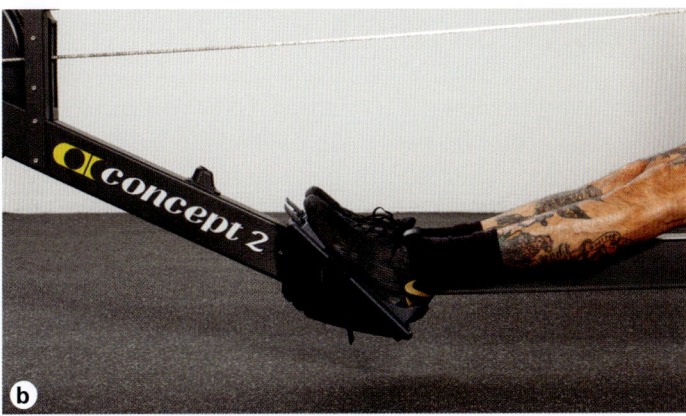

Pulling on the Straps

Pulling on the foot straps (see figure 4.5) typically happens at the finish of the stroke when you're using the straps to hold yourself in a hinged back position. This happens when there is a lack of core engagement at the finish. When you pull the straps, the tibialis anterior activates, which can cause shin or ankle pain. Additionally, you will feel tightness in the hip flexor muscles, typically caused by pulling on the straps to originate the recovery sequence or pulling yourself back to the catch position. Over time, this can cause back, hip, or groin pain from the psoas being overworked.

The best drill to fix this error is the strapless rowing drill found on page 53, with a focus on relaxing the ankles and keeping the toes in touch with the foot stretcher throughout the stroke.

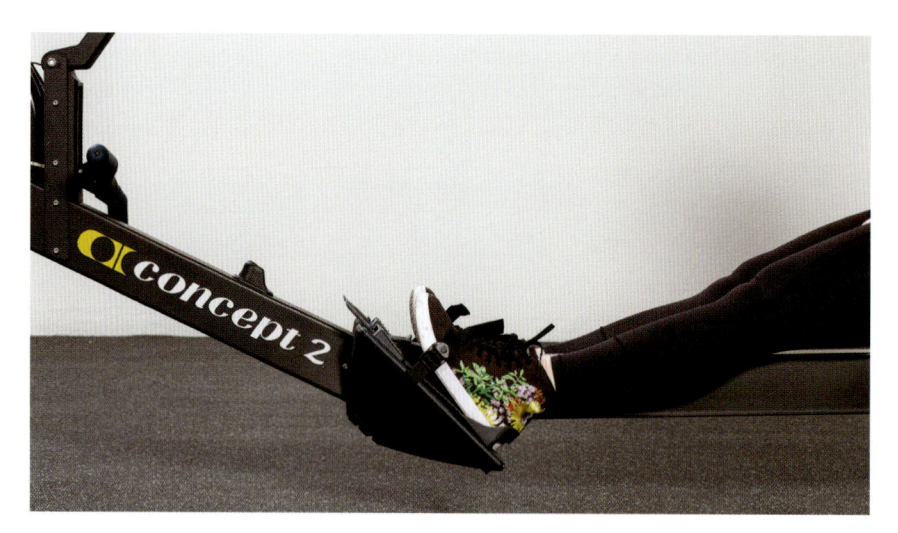

FIGURE 4.5 Pulling on the foot straps.

Excessive Layback or Overreaching

When you're looking for length in your stroke, you may surrender connection at both the catch and the finish by leaning beyond the one o'clock position in the finish or overreaching at the catch (figure 4.6). Excessive layback puts the lower back in an extended position, resulting in a lack of connection with both the abdominal wall and the lats. Without these muscles active, you lose connection to the core and the machine. This will increase the incidence of injuries to the lower back. Body awareness when fixing this error is critical. Setting up a recording device to record the stroke from a lateral viewpoint will help you spot any excessive layback. The strapless rowing drill on page 53 will help eliminate this error by forcing you to stop before laying back too far; otherwise, your feet will not stay in place!

Overreaching occurs when you try to extend your reach too far to increase your stroke length (figure 4.6), thus breaking the connection between the hips and shoulders that comes from posture. This can result in a loss of leverage and an inability to generate sufficient power. It can also put excessive strain on the back and shoulders, increasing the risk of injury to those areas. Posture is crucial to fixing this error. You should aim to keep your shoulders relaxed and your arms extended in a straight line with your torso, rather than reaching forward with your arms.

> **KEY POINT**
>
> To avoid overreaching, aim to keep your shoulders relaxed and your arms extended in a straight line with your torso rather than reaching forward with your arms.

A great drill to fix overreaching is the catch hold drill.

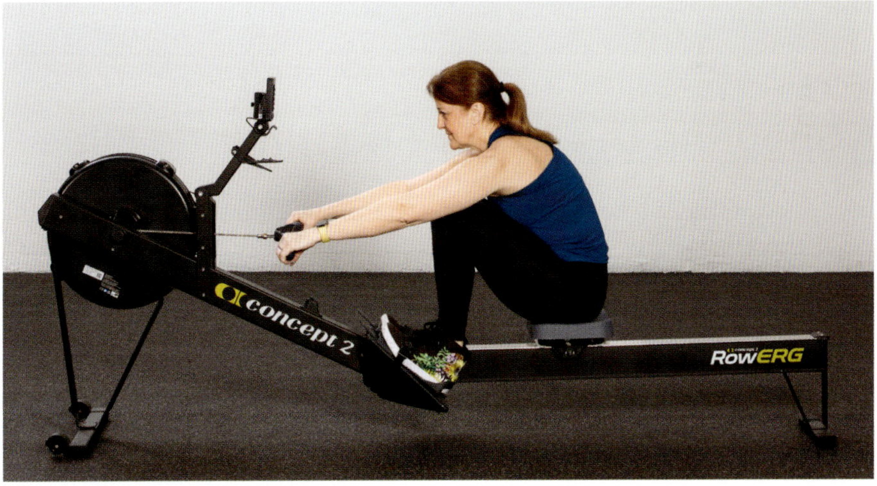

FIGURE 4.6 Overreaching at the catch.

CATCH HOLD DRILL

This drill will help you recognize the feeling of a tight and active catch.

- Find a strong catch position: vertical shins, seat six to eight inches from the feet, hips behind the shoulders, core engaged, arms reaching forward, and the handle hanging heavy in the fingertips with the pinkies at the edge (see photo).
- Hold this position for two minutes. Focus on your posture and the full engagement of the lats and core. You will NOT be comfortable!

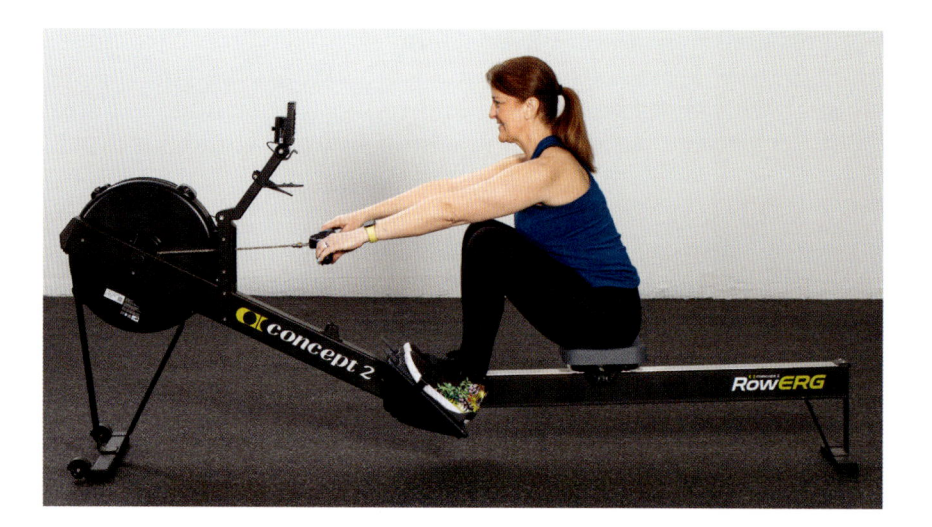

Shooting the Tail or Shooting the Slide

When driving back from the catch to the finish, the seat and the handle should move together. Sitting tall with relaxed shoulders and engaging the lats, rhomboids, and erector spinae muscles will connect the seat to the handle. Without this core engagement, the strong leg drive will send the seat back before the handle (figure 4.7).

When this error happens, it causes a loss of power at the hips because the power from the leg drive doesn't transfer to the handle. It also puts considerable pressure on the lower back. Fixing this error is as simple as activating all the muscles in your core. By tightening the muscles in the abdominal wall and depressing your shoulder blades down your back to activate the lats, you'll create the stability in the torso that is needed to keep the handle moving with the seat.

An effective drill to fix this error is the heavy handle drill (see page 51), as well as focusing on finding your core connection.

Common Errors in Rowing   **57**

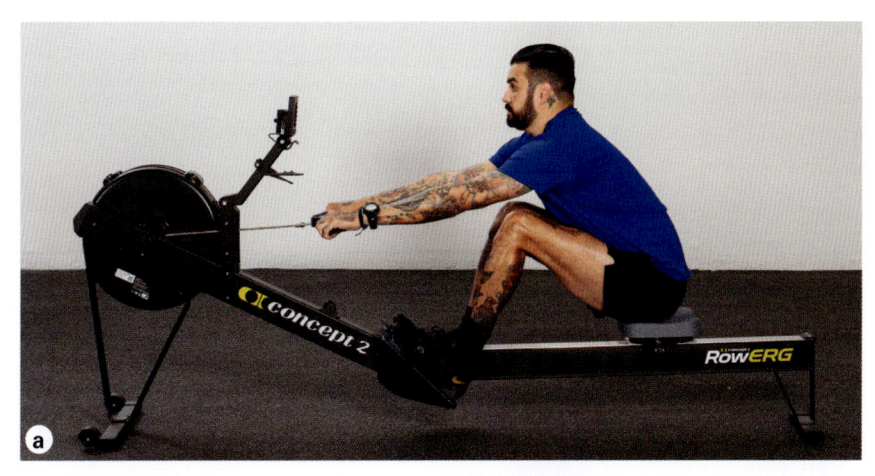

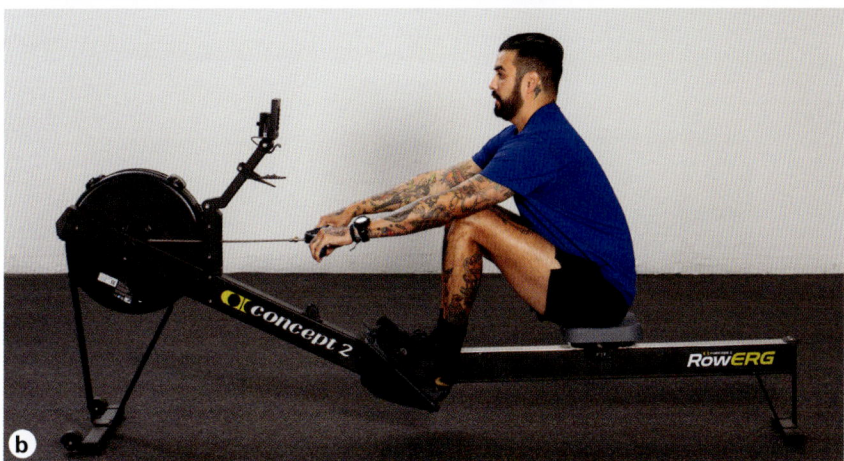

FIGURE 4.7 Without core engagement, you'll "shoot the tail," or send the seat back before the handle *(a)*. In a good stroke, the core is braced and allows you to bring the handle with you when the seat moves. The seat and handle should always move together on the drive *(b)*.

Not Using Ratio or Enough Leg Drive

The legs are the powerhouse of the stroke! Not using enough leg drive results in less power. If you rely too heavily on your arms and upper body to generate power, you will not use the full potential of your leg muscles. Additionally, if the drive and recovery have the same timing and the ratio of the stroke isn't 2:1 or 3:1, the lack of drive will result in a higher split or lower wattage.

Fixing this error will open doors to lower splits and stronger overall conditioning. You can use the legs only pick drill found on page 46 to assist in finding leg drive. Another great drill to fix this error is the low stroke rate drill, which allows you to focus on a stronger leg drive.

LOW STROKE RATE DRILL

Core engagement is important to keep the lower back strong and safe. Rowing with intensity (low splits) at low stroke rates (see photos) will teach you how to generate a strong drive by reinforcing the length of the recovery. This is a great drill to use if you have a rushed recovery or 1:1 ratio (the drive and recovery are the same length).

- Start in a strong catch position with good posture, with the shoulders in front of the hips and arms reaching forward. Engage the lats and brace the belly. Use the monitor to get a visual representation of stroke rate and split time.
- Holding 16 to 18 strokes per minute, row with the intent to drop your split time.
- Maintain a ratio count of one on the drive and four to six on the recovery.

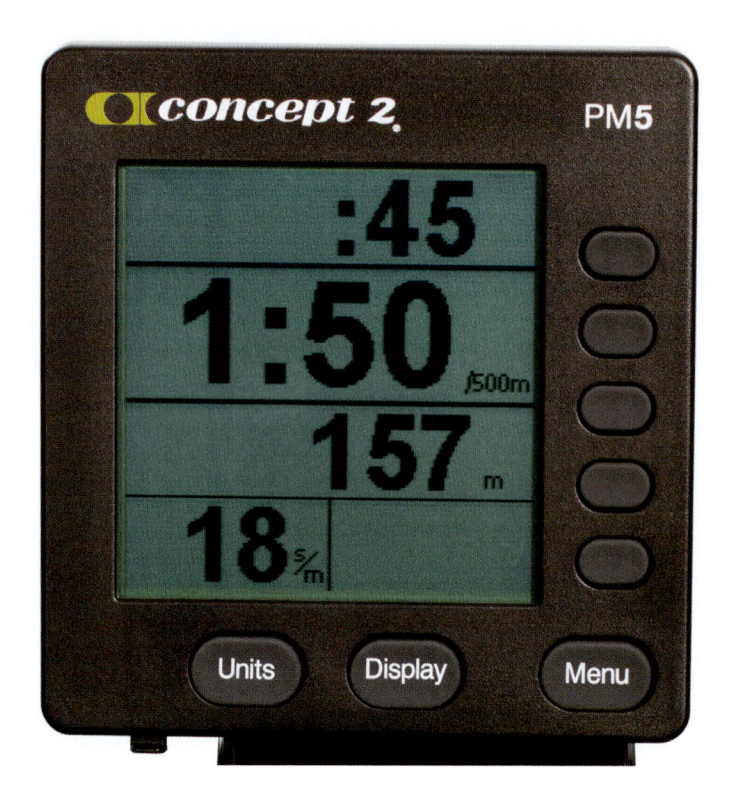

An effective way to understand what errors might be holding you back from a powerful stroke is to record yourself with a simple smartphone video. Set up your smartphone to record your stroke in slow motion. A slow-motion video will allow you to analyze each part of the stroke in pieces and identify any errors. Work through the recommended drills until you're satisfied that you've fixed your errors and are accessing the highest level of power in the stroke.

PART III

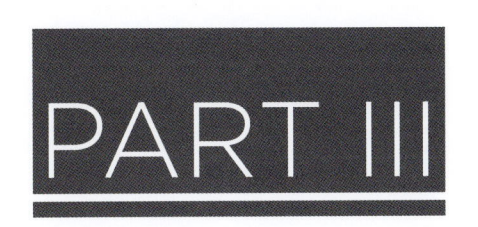

SAMPLE ROWING WORKOUTS AND STRETCHES

5

TYPES OF WORKOUTS

Though there are many nuanced approaches to training based on your goals, there are two dominant approaches to enhancing your overall physical performance both on and off the rowing machine: interval training and endurance training. These two training approaches will not only cater to the specific goals you may have but also induce physiological adaptations within the body. Whether you are a seasoned athlete or an aspiring fitness enthusiast, understanding the intricacies of endurance and interval training methodologies is helpful to get you closer to accomplishing your goals.

Endurance Versus High-Intensity Interval Training

Endurance training primarily targets the aerobic energy system, while traditional high-intensity interval training (HIIT training) works both the aerobic and anaerobic systems. It is important, however, to keep in mind that not all interval training needs to be high intensity. Intervals can have varying degrees of intensity. Interval training simply means pairing bursts of heavier effort with lighter recovery efforts. A workout in which you're shifting from 40% effort to 95% effort is very different from a workout in which you're shifting from 20% effort to 70% effort. Endurance training and high-intensity interval training can incorporate intervals, depending on how they're programmed and executed.

> **KEY POINT**
> Endurance training primarily targets the aerobic energy system, while traditional HIIT training works both the aerobic and anaerobic systems.

Aerobic exercise uses oxygen, and anaerobic exercise does not use oxygen. This means that aerobic exercise relies on oxygen as fuel or energy for the body to sustain the effort for prolonged periods. How long should workouts last to capture aerobic benefits? Typically, endurance workouts use sustained efforts at about 50% max heart rate for at least

> ## Workout Terminology
>
> Included here are a few key terms that are important to understand as we dive deeper into these specific training styles
>
> - *Cardiorespiratory endurance:* ability of the heart and lungs to produce oxygen for muscles during a sustained exercise bout
> - *Intervals:* cycles of high-intensity efforts and recovery periods during a workout
> - *Interval training:* training that cycles through high-intensity efforts and recovery periods, relying on both the aerobic and anaerobic energy systems
> - *Endurance training:* training that focuses on sustained efforts over a longer period, primarily targeting the aerobic energy system
> - *Muscular endurance:* muscles' ability to sustain prolonged, increasing tension and activation over time
> - *Aerobic energy system:* long-term energy production with oxygen, primarily used in endurance training, secondarily in interval training
> - *Anaerobic energy system:* short-term energy production without the need for oxygen during anaerobic exercise, typically used in high-intensity interval training (HIIT)
> - *Fast-twitch muscle fibers (type II):* quick-contracting muscle fibers, primarily involved with high-intensity interval training and explosive efforts
> - *Slow-twitch muscle fibers (type I):* slow-contracting muscle fibers, primarily involved with longer endurance-style training at a sustainable intensity
> - $\dot{V}O_2 max$: measure of aerobic capacity—commonly called the size of your aerobic engine—maximum rate of oxygen consumption during high-intensity exercise.
> - *Lactate threshold:* point at which lactic acid builds up in the blood.
> - *EPOC (excess post-exercise oxygen consumption):* increased oxygen consumption after intense exercise.

30 minutes. Over time, with training, you can increase your aerobic capacity, which means you'll be able to maintain a more elevated effort for a longer period. If you're just getting started on your exercise journey and it seems daunting to exercise for 30 minutes, begin with less and build up from there.

Anaerobic exercise does not use oxygen to supply energy; instead, it uses energy already stored in your muscles and burns that off during the typically shorter bouts of activity. Why are anaerobic exercise efforts shorter? Because you only have so much energy stored in your muscles, once that is used up, you'll need to recover and restore your breathing and oxygen supply. Through training, you can increase your anaerobic capacity or $\dot{V}O_2$max, which essentially means your body and muscles can sustain higher-intensity efforts without oxygen for a longer period. Anaerobic training can also elicit EPOC in your body, which is commonly referred to as the afterburn effect. EPOC stands for excess post-exercise oxygen consumption, which essentially is the amount of oxygen consumption needed to repair and restore the body back to homeostasis. The higher the intensity of the workout, the more oxygen needed after the workout to allow for the body's core temperature to cool, thus eliciting a higher caloric burn post workout. This is an important exercise factor for anyone who has the goal of losing weight and burning fat.

In building your anaerobic capacity, you're essentially building your body's lactate threshold, or your body's tolerance to the buildup of lactic acid. In simple terms, when your muscles have run out of oxygen supply to use as energy, they begin to burn off carbohydrates into glucose (a type of sugar) to produce fuel. In this process of producing fuel from glucose, lactic acid begins to build. Once lactic acid builds, the body then distributes it into the bloodstream to be broken down. If you've ever performed high-intensity exercise and felt a burning sensation in your muscles, you likely had lactic acid building up due to the lack of oxygen as fuel. As you train the anaerobic system, you build up your lactate threshold, allowing you to sustain higher intensity efforts for longer. True anaerobic intensities can typically last from 10 to 90 seconds depending on your conditioning; however, over time, you can improve your anaerobic capacity to increase the time sustained. You may wonder: How can I possibly get my heart rate up high enough in such a short interval of time to max out my anaerobic threshold? Rowing is a great answer! Because rowing works so many muscles at once and all the larger muscle groups, your working muscles demand more support from your heart and lungs. You will find that if you're rowing with strong power, you will be able to get your heart rate up very quickly. Rowing is commonly known as one of the most efficient workouts you can do, and working so many muscles at once is a big factor in its efficiency.

$\dot{V}O_2$max and Exercise

Our bodies rely heavily on oxygen throughout exercise, which leads us to the topic of $\dot{V}O_2$max. What is $\dot{V}O_2$max and why should we care about it? Your $\dot{V}O_2$max is your body's maximum amount of oxygen intake during exercise. As we know, oxygen is the fuel for aerobic exercise, so by improving your $\dot{V}O_2$max, you'll expand your body's oxygen intake, allowing for more endurance and stamina at any intensity level, low, moderate, or high. Improving your $\dot{V}O_2$max will leave you less winded when you perform ordinary daily activities like walking up stairs or chasing after a toddler. High-intensity interval training seems to be the most common and possibly the most effective way to increase your $\dot{V}O_2$max, though aerobic endurance training also contributes to improvements as well.

> **KEY POINT**
>
> By improving your $\dot{V}O_2$max, you'll expand your body's oxygen intake, allowing for more endurance and stamina at any intensity level, low, moderate, or high.

Type I and Type II Muscle Fibers

Let's not forget that your musculature and strength play a large role in your body's ability to excel at endurance-style workouts and power-based, high-intensity efforts. Our body is made up of type I and type II muscle fibers. Type I muscle fibers, also known as slow-twitch or slow-oxidative muscles, have a high tolerance to fatigue. Type II muscle fibers, also known as fast twitch, are generally quicker to fatigue; however, they contract quickly with a high production of power. As your endurance improves, your type I muscle makeup is enhanced. As your speed and power improve, your type II muscle makeup is enhanced. It's important to consider your muscle makeup as you're training your body. Whether your goal is to build strength, power, or muscular endurance will dictate what type of exercises you do, the volume of exercise, and the intensity and duration.

> **KEY POINT**
>
> Type I muscle fibers, also known as slow-twitch or slow-oxidative muscles, have a high tolerance to fatigue. Type II muscle fibers, also known as fast twitch, are generally quicker to fatigue; however, they contract quickly with a high production of power.

Mental Component of Training

The final component of endurance training and interval training is one that many people don't consider: the mental component of strengthening aerobic capacity, endurance, and $\dot{V}O_2$max. Endurance training requires a different type of mental focus than high-intensity interval training. If you want to build your endurance, you'll need to get strong at keeping your mind focused for a longer period of time. You'll want to improve your ability to get in the zone and build consistency, not allowing external distractions and thoughts to sway your performance. There are different methods to improve your mental focus and game for endurance training. Some common techniques in cardiorespiratory training include using music, breathing techniques, and cadence or stroke count, as well as learning whether you are more effective when training with timed workouts or task-based workouts.

Music

When deciding which music to listen to while you train, some considerations may include the energy and tempo of the music. Though music is multifaceted, the energy of a song, as well as the tempo, could have a big impact on your performance. Many athletes listen to music with a specific tempo to allow them to stay focused and keep their pace by matching their cadence with the beat of the music, like a metronome.

Aside from music tempo, the energy of a song or playlist also matters. If you're doing an endurance workout that's longer, you may consider music that has a steady driving beat but not anything too intense because it will be important to maintain energy and not go out too quickly. If it's a short, interval-based workout, consider music that's a bit more upbeat and powerful to help motivate your intensity.

Breathing Techniques

Breathing should remain consistent in any movement you're performing. In rowing, athletes typically take two breaths per stroke if the intensity is above 50% and exhale at the finish. Maintaining consistent breathing patterns not only allows you to maintain your pace and oxygenate your body properly but also gives your mind something to focus on.

Stroke Count

In rowing, it's very common to count strokes. For an endurance piece, you may find success in counting 10 to 12 strokes for every 100 meters you need to row, because each stroke is *roughly* 10 meters per stroke, depending on your pacing. So, mentally, rather than thinking "I have 1,000 meters to go," you may do better with "I have 10 sets of 10 strokes to go" and count them down accordingly. In addition to counting strokes for endurance workouts, it is very common for rowers to leverage "power 10s" in a race or a shorter workout. In a power 10, you row 10 strokes with a bit more intensity, and you typically dedicate them to someone or something to provide additional motivation. Some examples may be rowing 10 harder strokes for your coach, 10 harder strokes focusing on your leg drive, or 10 harder strokes to beat your opponent if you're in a race. Runners will often use the scenery around them, like running to a light pole or to the end of the street, to help compartmentalize the distance. On a fixed rowing machine, we don't have that same scenery, so we can leverage stroke count to help us get through the workout.

Training to Time or Task

In regard to choosing workouts or training for a race or event, it is important to understand yourself as an athlete to know what motivates you most. For example, rowing for a two-minute interval for maximum distance and the task of rowing 500 meters as quickly as possible may be comparable in terms of effort and length; however, one might allow you to focus and work harder due to the varying approaches. Some people may be more motivated by time, whereas others may need to see the meters ticking down in a 500-meter interval to maximize their power and speed. Other examples of task-based exercise are rowing or running for a specific calorie count or doing a specific number of repetitions of a series of movements. Typically in a task-based workout, once the task is complete, the workout is done. This is a motivating factor for many to push a bit harder. If the goal is to expand your anaerobic capacity leveraging high-intensity intervals, you'll need to improve your ability to go into the "pain cave" and go "into the red." Naturally, our bodies want to avoid discomfort; however, we need to learn how to stay in the discomfort for longer in order to maximize our results. For some, thinking "I only have to row for two minutes" will allow them to maximize their intensity and discomfort, which will result in more growth. For others, thinking "As soon as these 500 meters are done, then I can rest" elicits a better response in their body. Listening to your body and understanding what your body needs to perform at its highest is key, especially in a rowing or fitness race. As an example, the 2,000-meter row (2K) is the most tested distance in the sport of rowing. It is no joke. It requires strategy, a strong start, steady patience at times, and the ability to know the exact moment when it's time to "drop the hammer" and go all out. Many people will misjudge their body's ability in a 2,000-meter row and go all out too soon, which means they end up slowing down because they've completely burned their energy system and capacity. This is called *flying and dying* in the rowing community. The mind is a powerful thing in training, workouts, and races. While not every workout needs to be an all-out effort, learning what you need to find peak focus during exercise will help you maximize your results and time spent.

When approaching any workout on the rowing machine, regardless of the goal, there are a few additional factors to consider. Your ability to produce power in your stroke and control your cadence for efficiency is just as important as your ability to sustain strong cardiorespiratory efforts or have an effective mental strategy. The way you begin and end your workouts will also have a significant impact on the effectiveness of the workout, as well as your physical longevity and ability to recover between workouts. In the next chapter, we'll dive into productive warm-up and cool-down exercises for a rowing-based workout.

6

WARM-UP AND COOL-DOWN

Many people skip their warm-up and cool-down in their daily workout routine, which is unfortunate because they are so important to the success of your overall training. Your warm-up, if done well, should increase your mind–body connection as well as prepare your muscles to perform better in the workout ahead. Warming up means literally warming up your body. Your body temperature rises, and your blood begins to flow, carrying oxygen to your muscles. But that's not all—a good warm-up will also prepare your body for movement, so you get your body into safer, stronger positions for your workout. Think of it as movement prep.

> **KEY POINT**
>
> Your warm-up, if done well, should increase your mind–body connection as well as prepare your muscles to perform better in the workout ahead.

Here's an example: If you're about to do deadlifts, you might warm up the hip hinge movement pattern and loosen up the necessary muscles to allow your body to get into the best hip hinge prior to your deadlifts. It makes sense, right? First perfect the movement pattern without weight or resistance, then add load. This is especially important if you have any tightness in your muscles or restrictions in joint mobility that may prevent your body from getting into the best position.

Another example is preparing your body for an overhead press. If you're limited in shoulder mobility, you may need to spend some time at the beginning of your workout loosening up the latissimus dorsi (lats) and pectoralis muscles because those muscles could be restricting your ability to press successfully overhead. In this scenario, if someone is pressing overhead without properly aligned joints due to a lack of shoulder mobility, it could cause excess strain on the shoulder, resulting in a potential injury. However, if that same person spent time to warm up their shoulder press by loosening up the very muscles that could be tight and causing the lack of mobility, they would be more likely to reduce their risk of injury when performing the loaded overhead press because they'd perform the movement with better form.

Even something as low impact as rowing might require someone with tight hamstrings and glutei (glutes) to do some mobility work prior to jumping on the rower. Why? A hip hinge is the primary movement pattern for rowing. So, if you can't perform a proper hip hinge while standing, then there's a good chance you won't be able to perform a proper hip hinge while seated on the rower. Why is a proper hip hinge important for rowing? The hip hinge allows the hamstrings and glutes to be loaded properly as well as keeps the lumbar spine stabilized so that when you drive on the next stroke you're utilizing mostly the legs and core and the back stays protected. How do you know if you have mobility restrictions that may require additional warm up? First, let's look at the common mistakes in the hip hinge movement and what the root cause of the error could be (see table 6.1). Understanding this information will help you understand what your warm-up for a rowing workout should entail (also found in table 6.1).

You may be asking yourself why it's so important to perform hip hinges properly. Consider the load on your spine if your lumbar spine is rounded as you perform a heavy deadlift. Ouch! While the load of a rowing stroke is not as intense as a 300-pound deadlift, it still requires strong core engagement to stabilize the lumbar spine and activation of the legs to ensure the back isn't taking too much of the load. A proper hip hinge helps you to generate power efficiently and safely on the machine.

What we've learned so far is that hinging properly in your rowing stroke can help reduce the risk of injury. What else can hinging properly do? A proper hip hinge can improve muscle recruitment, so you get more out of your rowing. Right now, as you're reading this, go ahead and sit taller in your seat. What do you feel? More core activation? Yes. The same thing happens in your rowing when you sit taller. A strong hip hinge can also help recruit your hamstrings and glutes more. You'll feel the hamstrings lengthen on the recovery when rowing slowly. What happens when we lengthen our muscles? We load them. What happens when we load them? We use them, and they get stronger. Consider this: If you warm up your posterior chain (the muscular chain on the backside of your body) and overall hip hinge movement before rowing, you are likely going to recruit more muscles and move more safely, which results in a more impactful workout, driving more results.

> ### KEY POINT
> If you warm up your posterior chain (the muscular chain on the backside of your body) and overall hip hinge movement before rowing, you are likely going to recruit more muscles and move more safely, which results in a more impactful workout, driving more results.

TABLE 6.1 Common Errors in Hip Hinge Movement Pattern and Corresponding Suggested Warm-Ups

Error	Possible root cause	Suggested warm-up
Flexion in the lumbar spine	This will typically occur if you lack proper body mechanics and begin to reach for the toes, which will cause you to round through your low back instead of hinging from your hips. Tight (overactive) hamstrings could also be the cause as this would limit your ability to hinge properly from the hip joint while maintaining a neutral spine.	The goal in this warm-up is to ensure your hip hinge body mechanics are correct as well as begin to lengthen through the posterior chain. 1. Grab a dowel rod or PVC! Perform 2 sets of 15 reps of dowel rod–assisted good mornings. 2. Take it to the wall! Stand about 1 foot from the wall and perform 2 sets of 15 reps of good mornings. Your goal is to tap your glutes on the wall. 3. Walk it out! Perform 2 sets of 15 reps of walkouts to begin lifting the heart rate while still reinforcing the proper hip hinge and lengthening through the posterior chain.
Extension in the lumbar spine	This is also known as an anterior pelvic tilt, or lumbar lordosis. This might be evidence of a weak core and overactive erector spinae muscles. Showing extension in the lumbar spine while performing a hip hinge could also simply be poor body mechanics in the initial movement of the hip hinge.	A warm-up of dynamic stretches to release the erector spinae would be 3 rounds of the following exercises: 1. Perform 15 reps of cat–cow. 2. Perform 15 reps of bird dogs (each side). 3. Perform 30 seconds of child's pose.
Flexion in the thoracic spine	Rounding of the upper back can often be due to muscle tightness in the chest (pectoralis muscles), lats, and underactive upper back muscles (rhomboids, trapezius). Assess your posture when you're standing upright. If you see rounding of the upper back, it could mean there is dysfunction, and you might want to consult a physical therapist for guidance.	A warm-up to open the chest and lats while activating the upper back would be performing 2 rounds of the following exercises: 1. Perform 15 reps of PVC or banded shoulder pass throughs. 2. Perform 15 reps of walkouts. 3. Perform 15 reps of high plank to downward dog. 4. Perform 15 reps of sphinx t-spine rotation (each side). 5. Grab a dowel rod! Perform 15 reps of dowel rod–assisted good mornings.

Warm-Up Exercises

The following warm-up exercises are designed to prepare your body for the movement pattern of rowing. Primarily they will focus on lengthening and warming up the posterior chain, mobilizing the hips as well as activating the core. Warming up properly for the rowing motion will allow for better body positioning in the catch position due to greater mobility and flexibility, resulting in more muscle activation and stronger power in the stroke.

DOWEL ROD–ASSISTED GOOD MORNINGS

INSTRUCTIONS

- Stand tall with your feet hip-width apart, with a slight bend in the knees. Place a dowel rod behind your head between your shoulders and hold the rod with both hands *(a)*.
- As you exhale, hinge forward at the hips, keeping the spine long and chest lifted. Hinge until you feel a stretch in the hamstrings *(b)*.
- As you inhale, return to standing while keeping the spine long.
- Repeat for the desired number of repetitions.

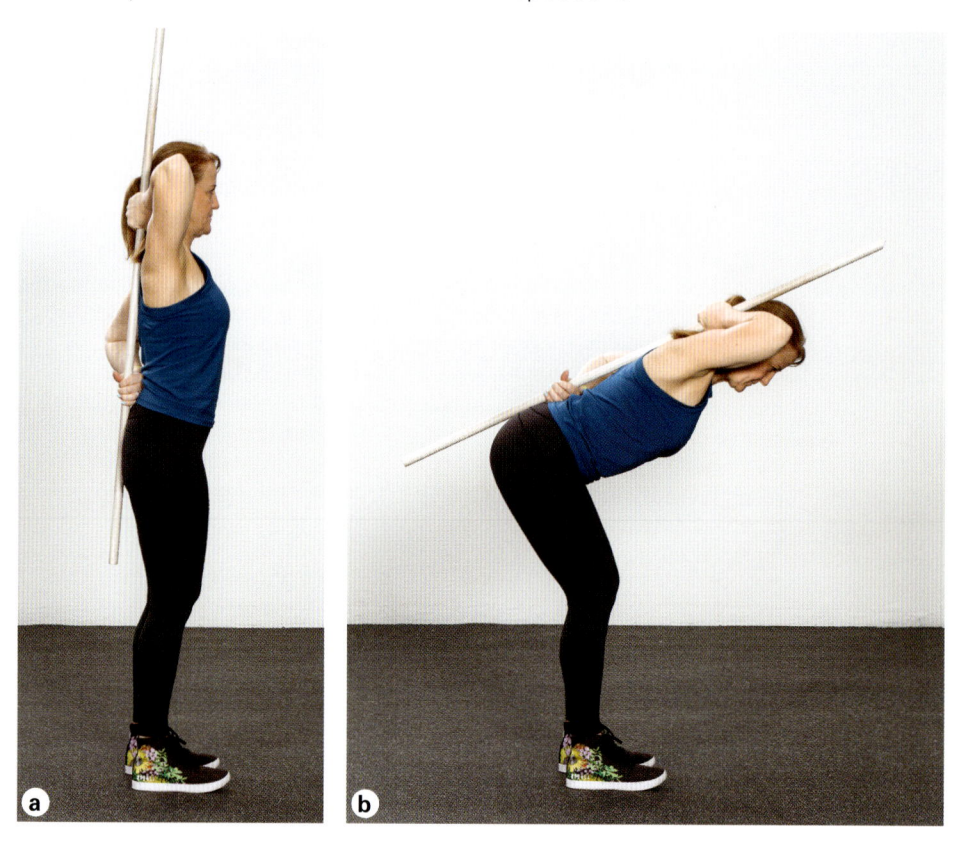

Warm-Up and Cool-Down 75

GOOD MORNINGS

INSTRUCTIONS

- Begin with your feet hip-width apart, with a slight bend in the knees. Your hands can be behind your head, on your hips, or behind your low back *(a)*.
- Hinge your upper body at the hips while maintaining a neutral spine and braced core.
- Hinge until you feel a slight stretch of the hamstrings or until the body is parallel (or as close to parallel as you can get while still maintaining a neutral spine) to the ground, then return to an upright standing position *(b)*.

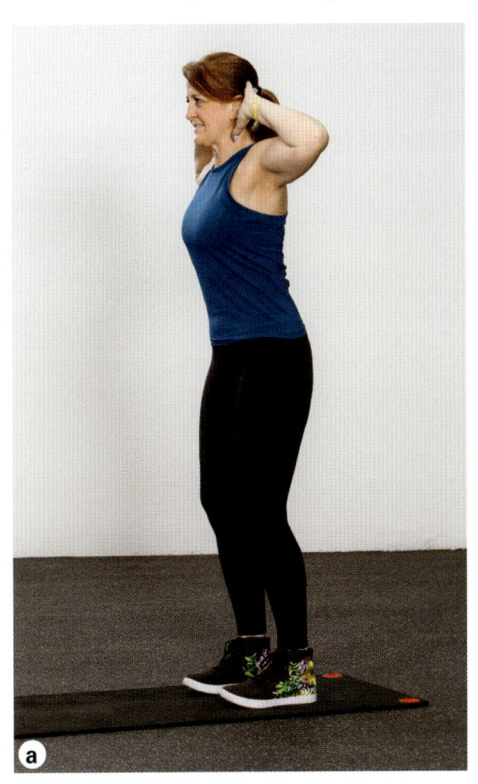

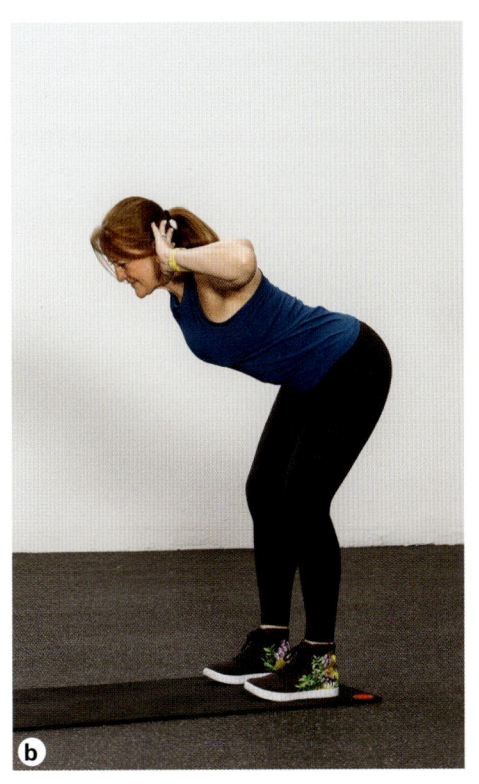

WALKOUTS

INSTRUCTIONS

- Begin with your feet about shoulder-width apart, with a slight bend in the knees. Hinge your upper body at the hips while maintaining a neutral spine and braced core *(a)*.
- Reach your hands to the ground and walk them out to a high plank position *(b)*.
- Hold the plank for a few seconds, then send the hips up to the sky and slowly walk the hands back into the feet.
- Bring the body up to a standing position by reversing the action of how you got down.
- Repeat for the desired number of repetitions. Aim to keep your legs as straight as possible during this exercise to feel a stronger stretch in the hamstrings.
- If you're looking to amplify muscle recruitment and increase the heart rate, a good option is to add a push-up. In this movement, you simply walk your hands out to a high plank, perform a push-up, lowering the chest to the ground with the elbows at a 45-degree angle to the body, and then push the body back up to a high plank.
- From there, walk your body back to standing by reversing the action.

Warm-Up and Cool-Down

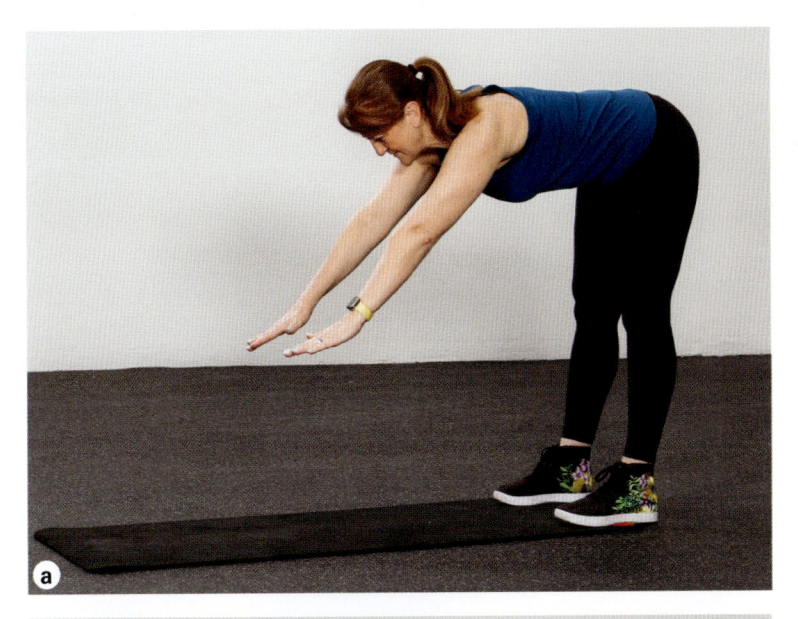

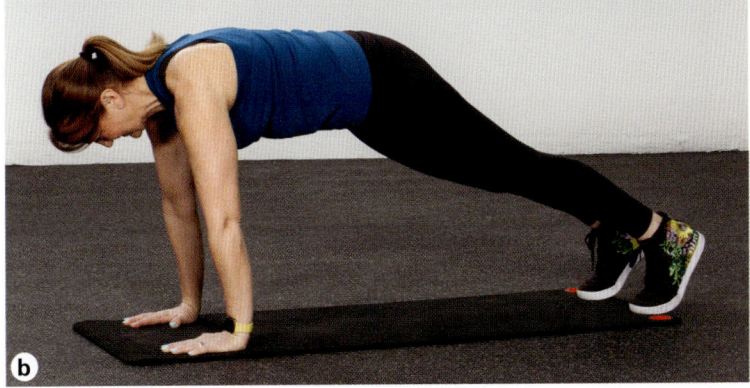

CAT-COW

INSTRUCTIONS

- Begin in a quadruped, or tabletop, position on your hands and knees.
- Flex through the spine, hollowing out the body as you tuck your chin into your chest *(a)*. This is the cat portion of the movement.
- From there, extend through the spine, pushing your ribs to the floor, and lift your head up to the sky *(b)*. This is the cow portion of the movement.
- Continue cycling between those two movements.

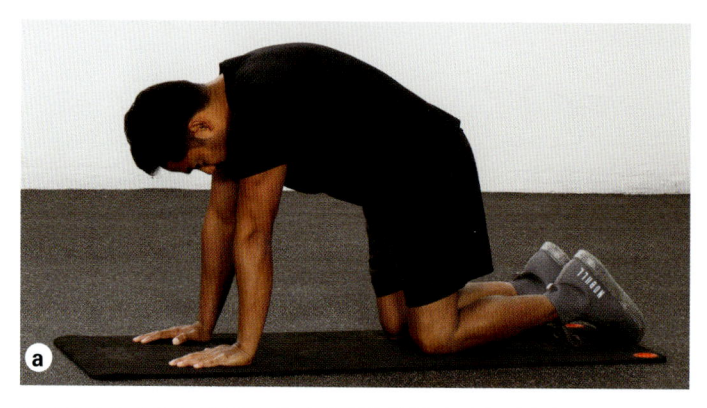

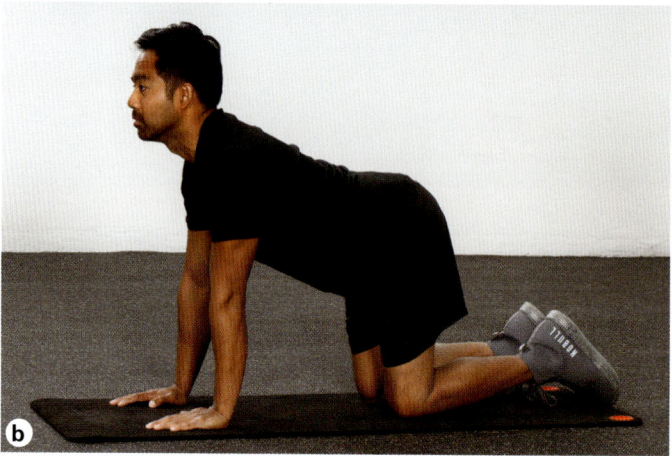

BIRD DOG

INSTRUCTIONS

- Begin in a quadruped, or tabletop, position on your hands and knees, with a 90-degree angle at your knees, hips, and shoulders *(a)*.
- Extend the left arm, reaching forward while simultaneously extending and reaching the right leg back *(b)*.
- Once you have fully extended the left arm and right leg, hold for a second, then bring them back to all fours and switch sides.
- If this exercise requires more core stability than your body is prepared for, modify it by lifting one arm or one leg at a time.
- If you want to increase the difficulty, stay on the same side for longer before switching arms and legs.

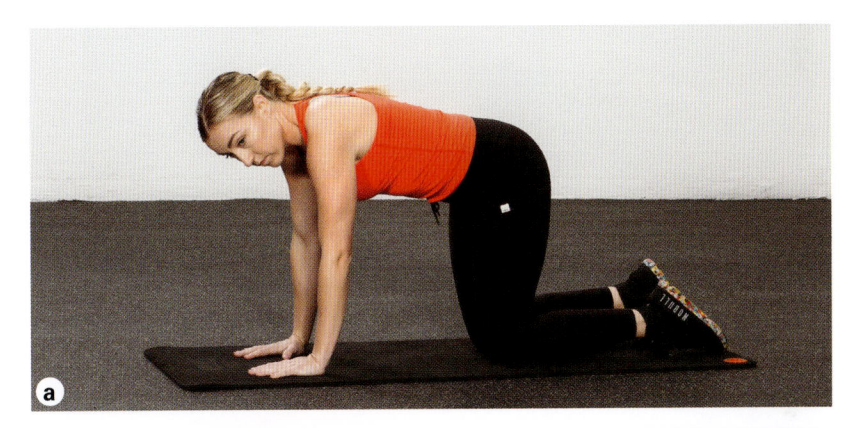

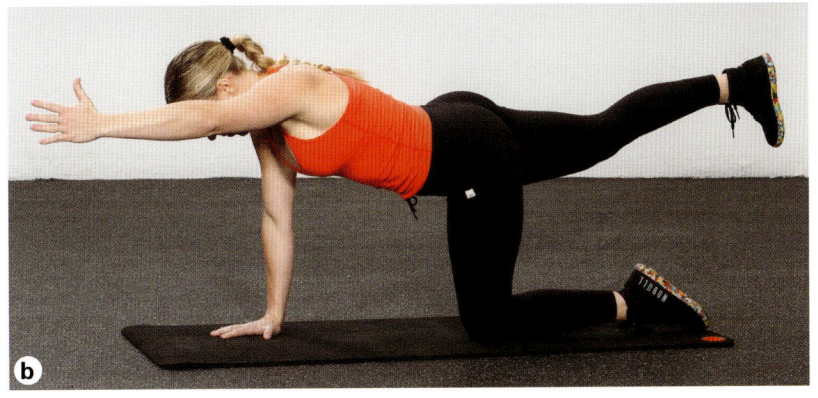

CHILD'S POSE

INSTRUCTIONS

- Begin in a quadruped, or tabletop, position on your hands and knees. Open your knees a bit wider, and shift your ankles and feet closer together.
- From there, shift the hips back so you're sitting on your ankles with your arms fully extended in front of you on the ground.
- Hold this pose for about 30 seconds.

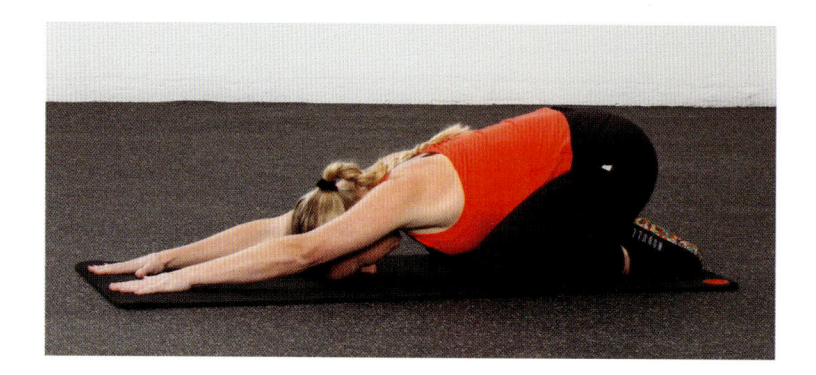

PVC OR BANDED SHOULDER PASS THROUGHS

INSTRUCTIONS

- Grab onto the PVC pipe or band, with each hand wider than the shoulders. Your arms should be fully extended and holding onto the PVC or band in front of your body, with the PVC or band resting down at your hips.
- Keep your arms fully extended as you pass the band or PVC over your head, behind you, and down to your hips.
- Reverse the movement as your arms pass back through above your head to land in the starting position down in front of your hips.
- If it's challenging to maintain straight arms through this movement, walk your hands wider on the PVC or band.

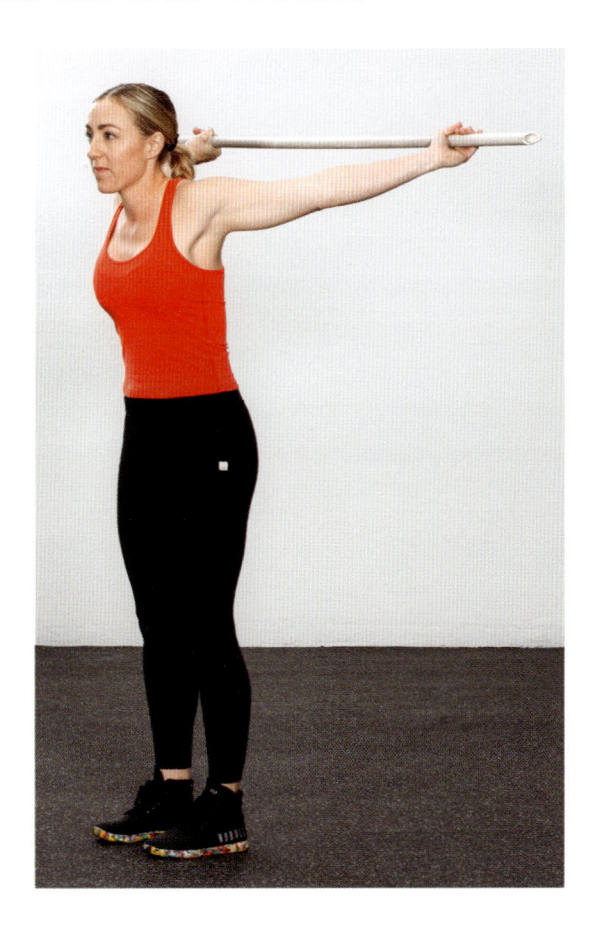

HIGH PLANK TO DOWNWARD DOG

INSTRUCTIONS

- Find a high plank position, with the hands pressing into the ground under the shoulders and the legs fully extended behind you. Press your heels back behind you *(a)*.
- From there, shift the hips up to a downward dog position, pressing the head through the arms and the heels into the ground *(b)*.
- Shift back to the high plank, and repeat.

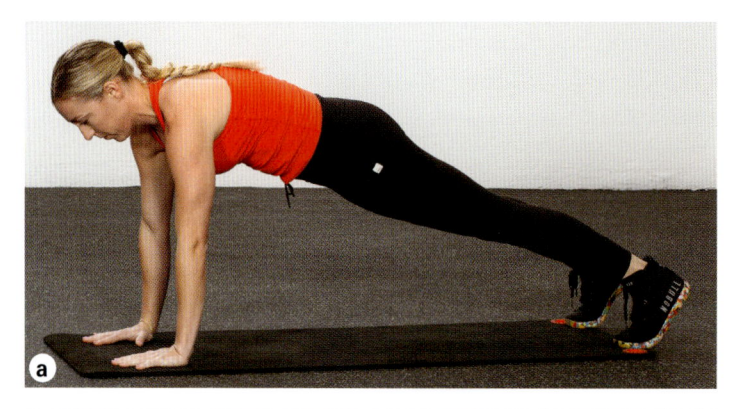

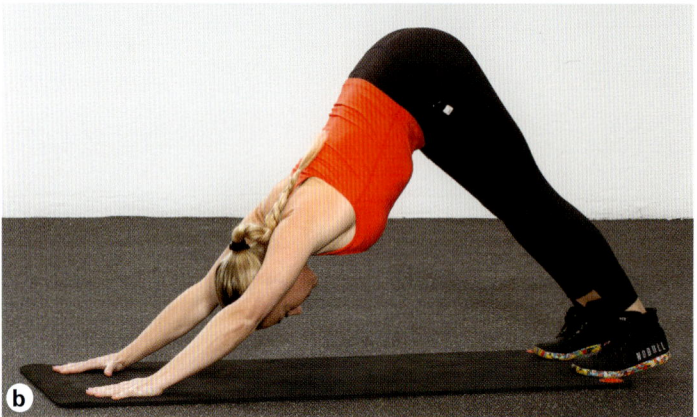

Warm-Up and Cool-Down 83

SPHINX T-SPINE ROTATION

INSTRUCTIONS

- Find a quadruped, or tabletop, position.
- From here, bend the left arm so the forearm is resting on the ground in front of you.
- Take the right hand and place it on your ear, bending the right arm with the palm against the back of your head and place that elbow resting on the ground in front of you *(a)*.
- With the right arm, rotate toward the right, opening the torso on the right side and feel the stretch in the thoracic spine *(b)*.
- From there, bring the right elbow that's up and bring it back to the starting point with the elbow resting lightly on the ground in front of you *(a)*.

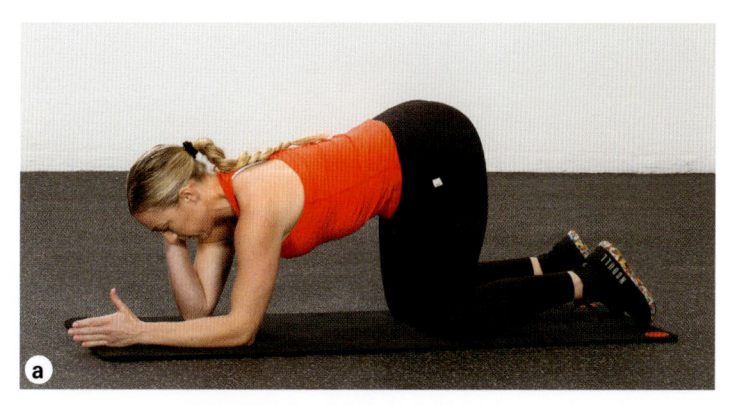

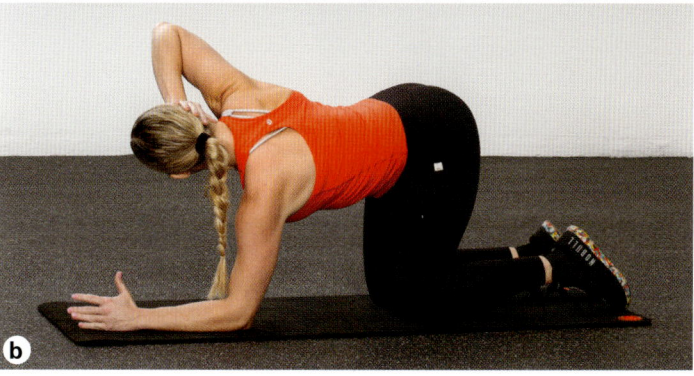

STANDING HIP CRADLE

INSTRUCTIONS

- Begin in a standing position. Shift your weight to one leg, then lift the other leg in front of you. With the opposite hand to the lifted leg, grab your ankle.
- With your other hand, hold the outside of your bent knee.
- Slightly rotate the lifted ankle toward the opposite side to feel a deeper stretch.
- Do this while balancing on the standing leg, then switch legs and arms.

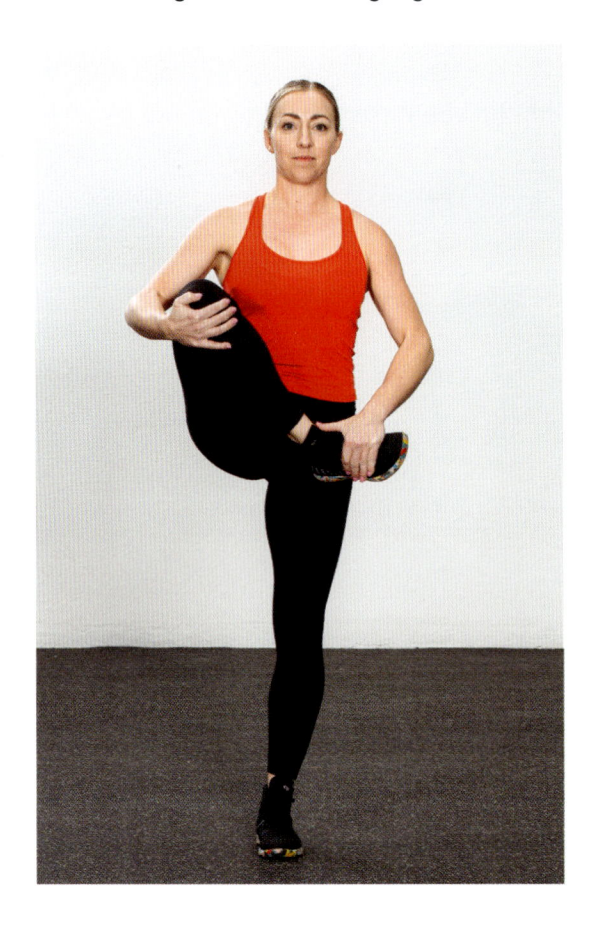

INCHWORMS

INSTRUCTIONS

- Start in a plank position, pull your hips to the sky, and walk your feet toward your hands, maintaining a long spine and straight legs.
- Walk in as far as possible for an effective hamstring stretch. From there, walk your hands out into a plank position.
- Repeat as desired. This movement does travel, so allow for ample space to move throughout the room.

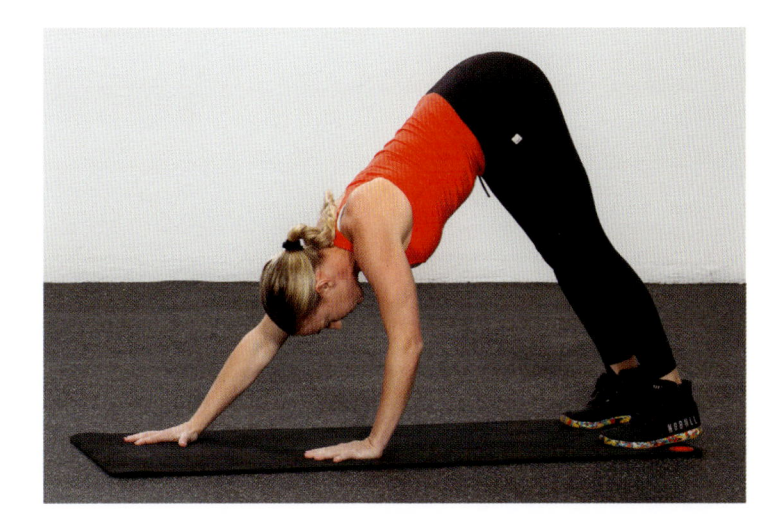

HAND RELEASE PUSH-UPS

INSTRUCTIONS

- Start facedown, with your legs extended and your hands just beneath your shoulders. Push yourself up to a high plank position *(a)*.
- Slowly lower yourself back to the floor, release your hands from the floor for two seconds *(b)*, then reconnect your hands to the floor and push yourself back to a plank.
- Focus on keeping a long spine and a straight line from your shoulders to your heels. To modify this movement, lower your knees to the ground.

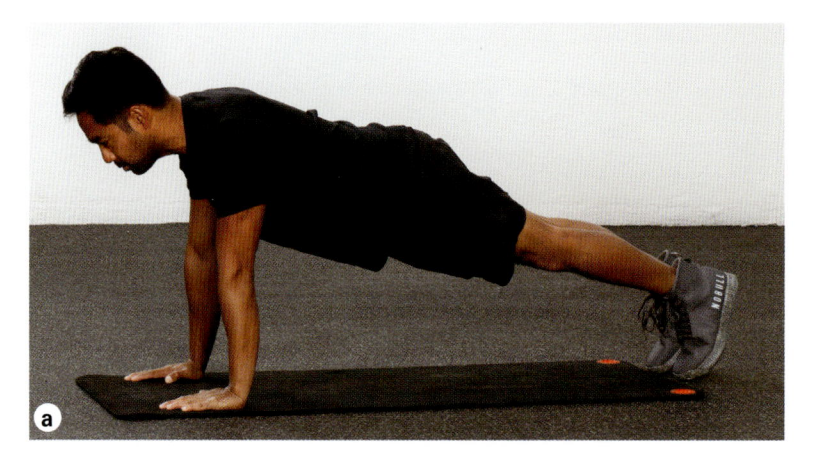

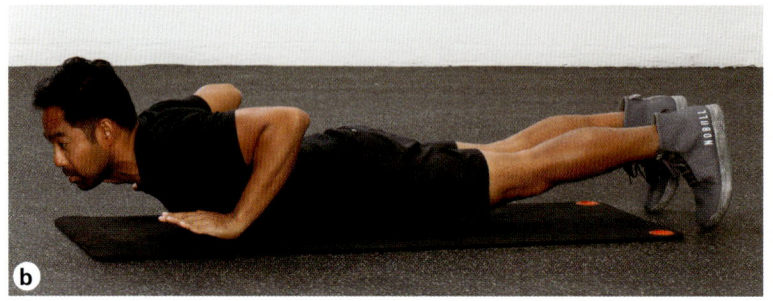

REVERSE LUNGE

INSTRUCTIONS

- Start with your feet hip-width apart, your torso upright, and your chest lifted with your shoulders back and down.
- Step straight back with your right foot, ensuring that you maintain the width of your stance and bend your knees while maintaining an upright positioning of the torso.
- Return to the starting position by pushing through the front heel and bringing your back foot to meet your front foot.
- Repeat on the opposite side.

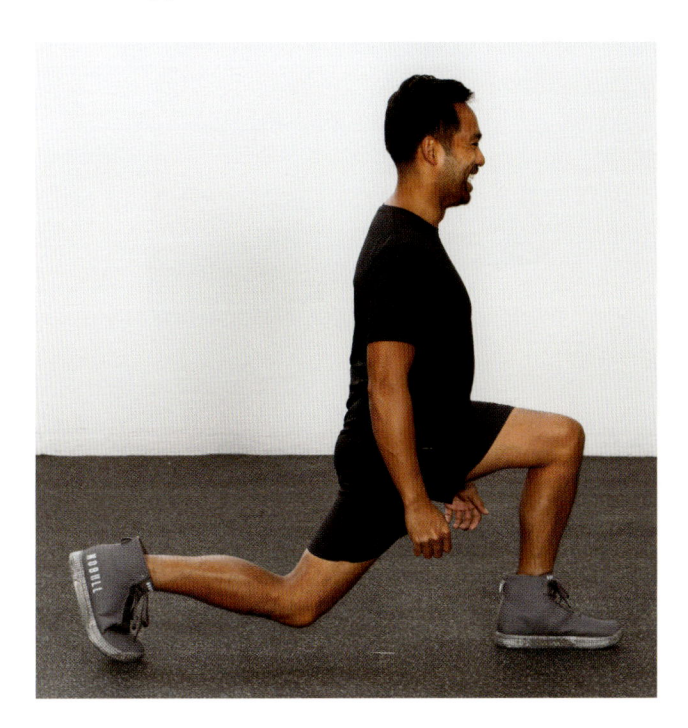

TIN SOLDIER

INSTRUCTIONS

- Start with your feet hip-width apart and your torso upright, with your arms hanging by your sides.
- Raise your left arm forward and concurrently bring your right leg up to meet your left fingers.
- Return to the starting position and repeat on the opposite side.

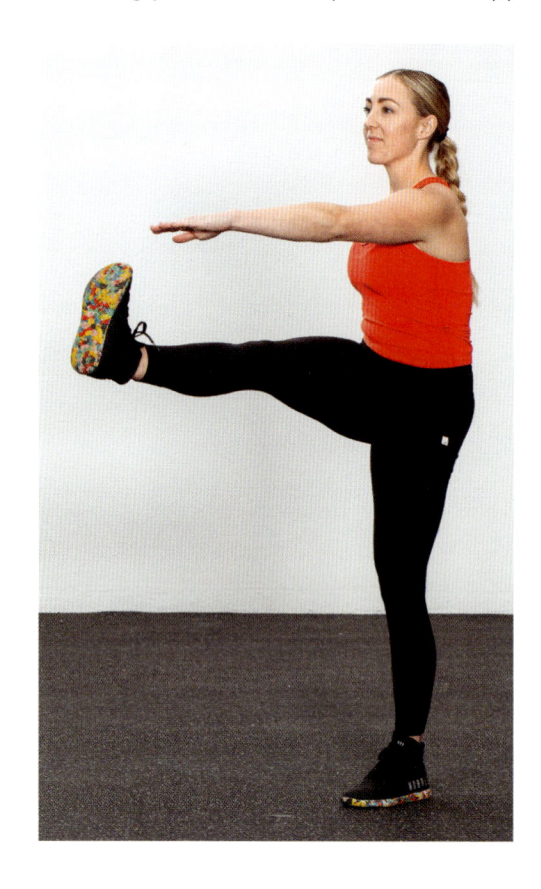

SQUAT STRETCH

INSTRUCTIONS

- Begin with your feet about shoulder width apart.
- Bend your knees slightly and hinge forward. Lightly grab your toes with your hands *(a)*. If you cannot reach your toes, you can reach for your shins.
- From this position, sink your hips down as low as you can, focusing on opening through the hips and keeping your chest lifted. In this position, you can use your elbows to press outward against your knees to open up the hips and feel a deeper stretch *(b)*.
- Keep your hands connected to your toes, and lift your hips as high as you can to feel a stretch in your hamstrings *(c)*.
- Shift back down, sinking your hips down as low as you can, focusing on opening through the hips and keeping your chest lifted. Cycle between this step and the previous one.

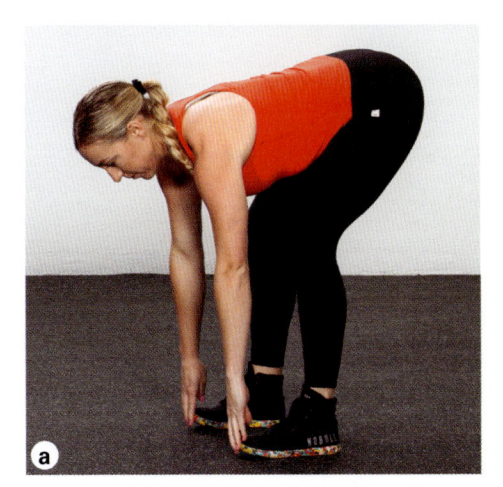

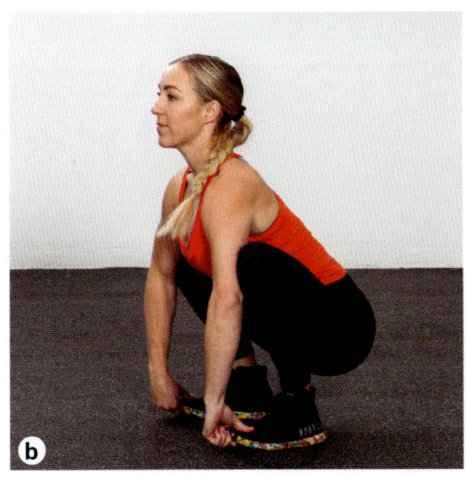

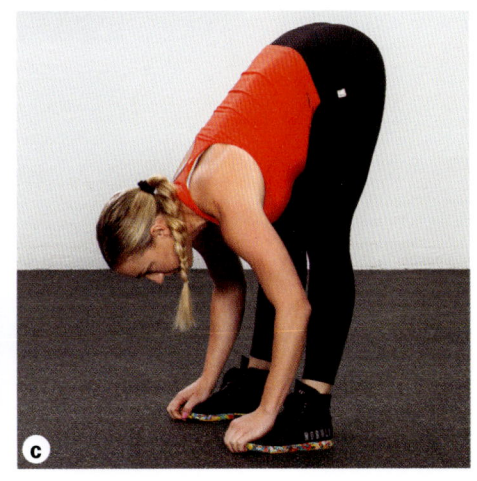

WALKOUT + PUSH-UP

INSTRUCTIONS

- Begin with your feet about shoulder-width apart, with a slight bend in the knees and your arms lifted overhead *(a)*.
- Hinge your upper body at the hips while maintaining a neutral spine and braced core.
- Reach your hands to the ground and walk them out to a high plank position, perform a push-up, lowering the chest to the ground with the elbows at a 45-degree angle to the body, and then push the body back up to a high plank *(b-c)*.
- From there, push the hips up as you walk the hands back closer to the feet, then bring the body up to a standing position by reversing the action of how you got down.

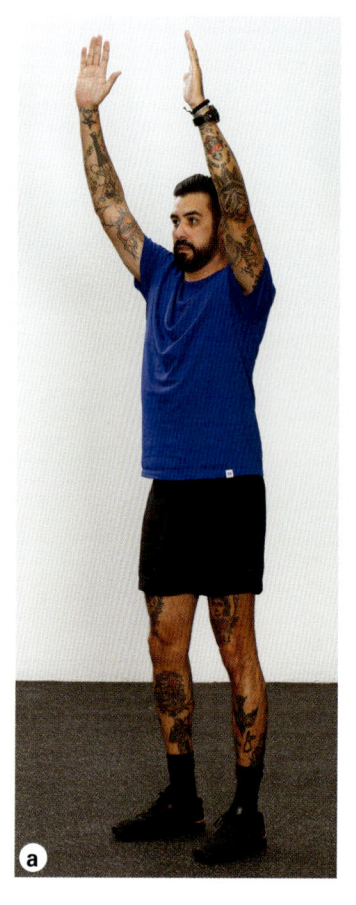

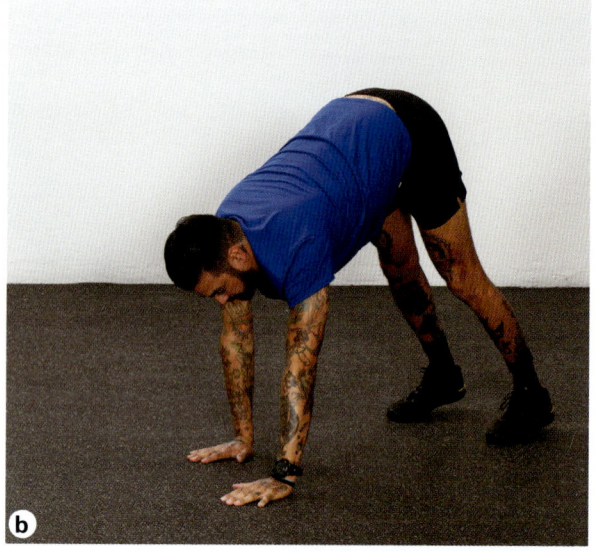

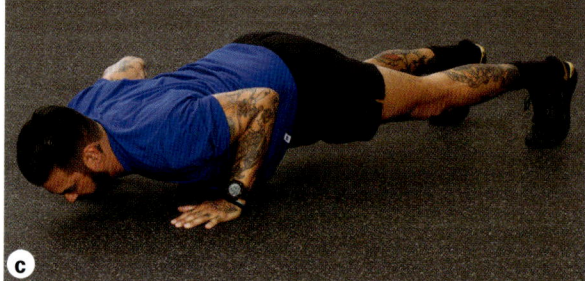

HIP ROTATION

INSTRUCTIONS

- Begin in a standing position with your feet hip-width apart and hands on your hips.
- Slowly shift your weight to the left leg and lift the right leg up to 90 degrees with a bent knee *(a)* and rotate outward *(b)* before bringing that leg back down.
- Shift the weight to the right leg and lift the left leg up to 90 degrees with a bent knee. Rotate the left leg outward and then bring it back down.
- Continue alternating legs and repeating this movement.
- Feel free to reverse the rotation and bring the leg out to in to maximize the mobility through the hip.

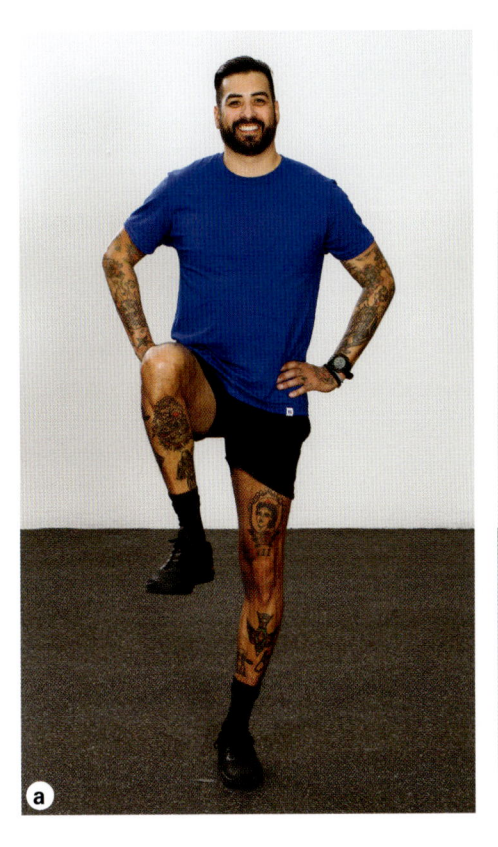

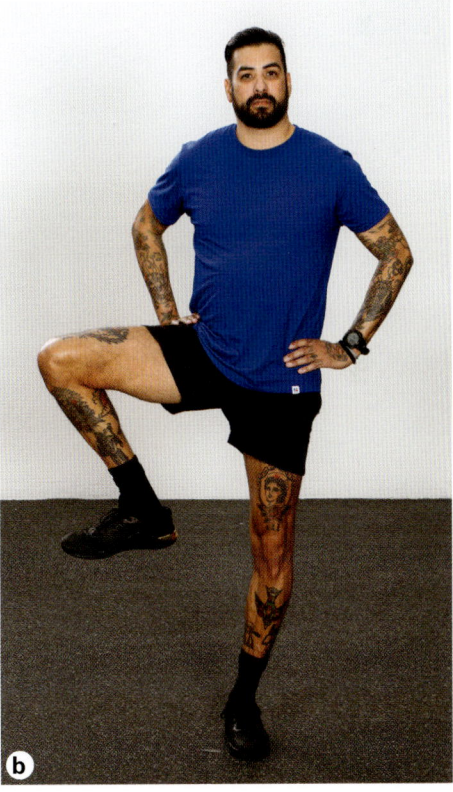

WORLD'S GREATEST STRETCH

INSTRUCTIONS

- Start in a high plank position and step your right foot to the outside of your right hand *(a)*.
- Keep your back leg extended, shift your weight, press your left hand into the ground, and rotate your torso to open your right hand to the sky *(b)*.
- Return your torso to the center. With your left arm straight and left hand pressing into the ground still, bend your right elbow, and send it down toward your right ankle, aiming to place the right forearm on the ground on the inside of your right ankle *(c)*.
- Return to the center position, step back into a high plank, and repeat on the other side.

Warm-Up and Cool-Down 93

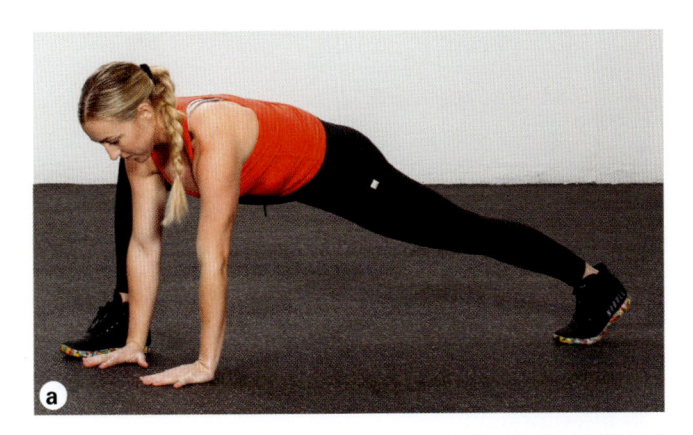

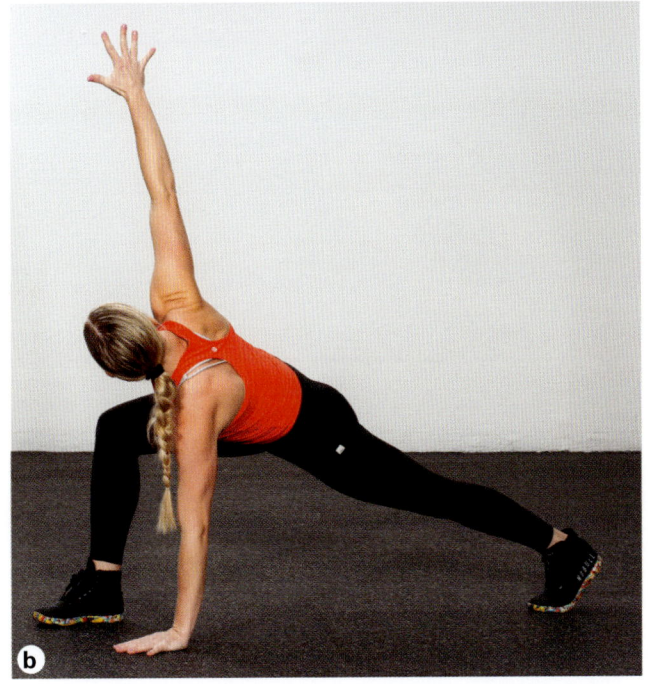

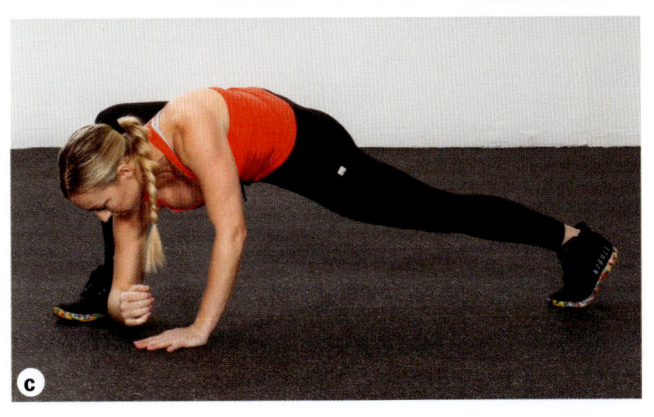

DYNAMIC HALF PIGEON

INSTRUCTIONS

- Start on your hands and knees, push yourself into a high plank position, and sweep your right leg forward so your right knee is just behind your right wrist. Drop the back leg down to rest on the floor behind you *(a)*. The closer your right foot is to your left inner thigh, the less you will feel the stretch in your right hip.
- Push your left hip toward the ground, lift your left arm off the floor, rotate, and reach under your right arm *(b)*. Repeat this for 15 to 30 seconds, then repeat on the other side.

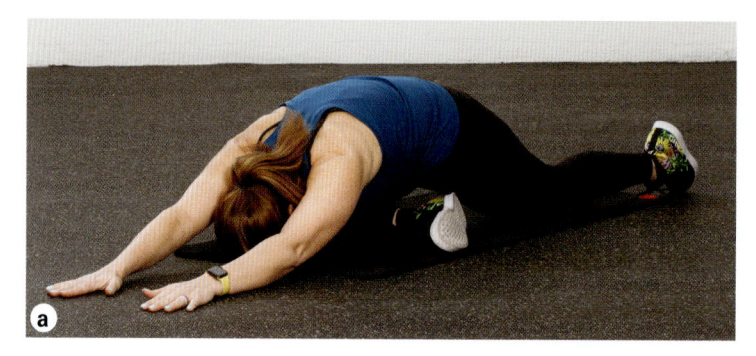

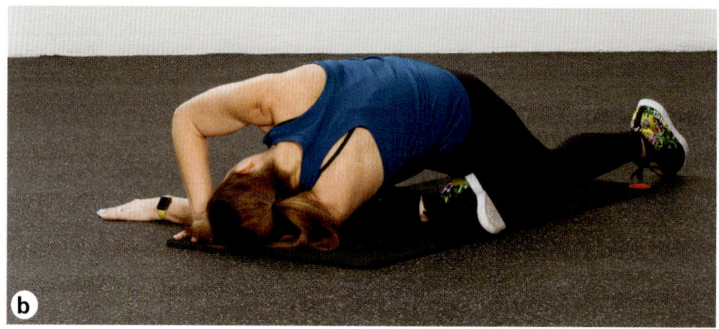

Dynamic Warm-Ups for Rowing Workouts

Let's dive into some off-rower warm-ups to prepare your body for a rowing workout. This section provides three dynamic body weight warm-ups for rowing workouts that open the posterior chain:

WARM-UP 1

Three rounds, 30 seconds each:

- Good mornings
- Standing hip cradles
- Inchworms
- Hand release push-ups

WARM-UP 2

Three rounds:

- 15 reverse lunges and tin soldiers (each leg)
- 10 squat stretches
- 5 walkout + push-ups

WARM-UP 3

Three rounds, 30 seconds each:

- Alternating reverse lunges and hip rotations
- World's greatest stretch left
- World's greatest stretch right
- Dynamic half pigeon

Rowing Warm-Ups for Rowing Workouts

These suggested rowing-based warm-ups will prepare the body for both a rowing workout and an off-the-rower workout. We start with traditional rowing warm-ups to prepare us for a rowing-based workout or simply the movement pattern of rowing, a hip hinge. In this section are two drill-based warm-ups that can be effective for any type of rowing workout, regardless of whether you're prepping your muscles for an endurance or interval-based rowing workout.

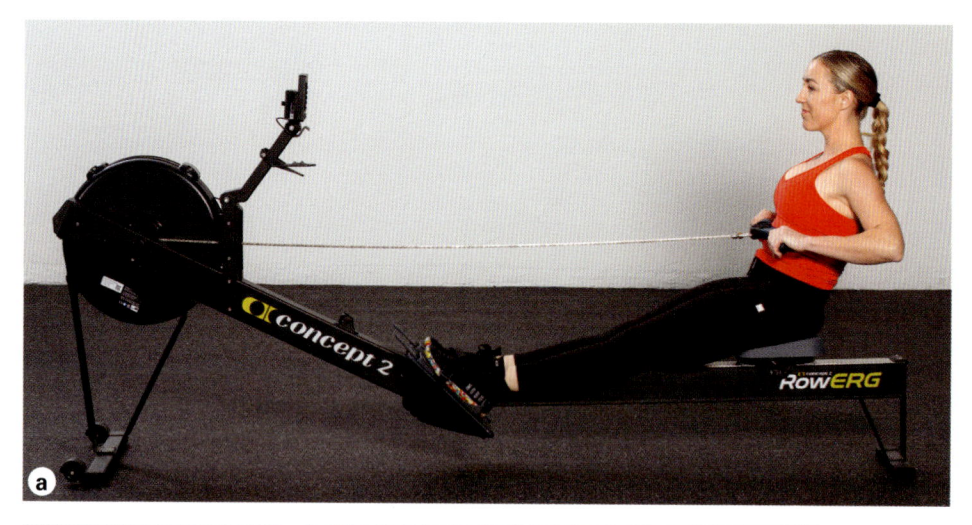

ARMS ONLY PICK DRILL

In rowing, a pick drill picks apart the stroke, piece by piece, to perfect, improve, and warm up each part of the stroke. These drills are often used when rowing on the water because they help you improve your stroke one section at a time. It is a great way to slowly begin to elevate your heart rate and warm up your muscles, all while reinforcing proper movement. This drill specifically focuses on the recovery sequence and control.

- Begin in the finish position, extending and flexing only the arms *(a* and *b)*.
- Add the upper body swing (hip hinge) so that the arms and body move forward and back *(c)*.
- Move into a half stroke (half the distance up the slide) *(d)*.
- Perform the full stroke *(e)*.

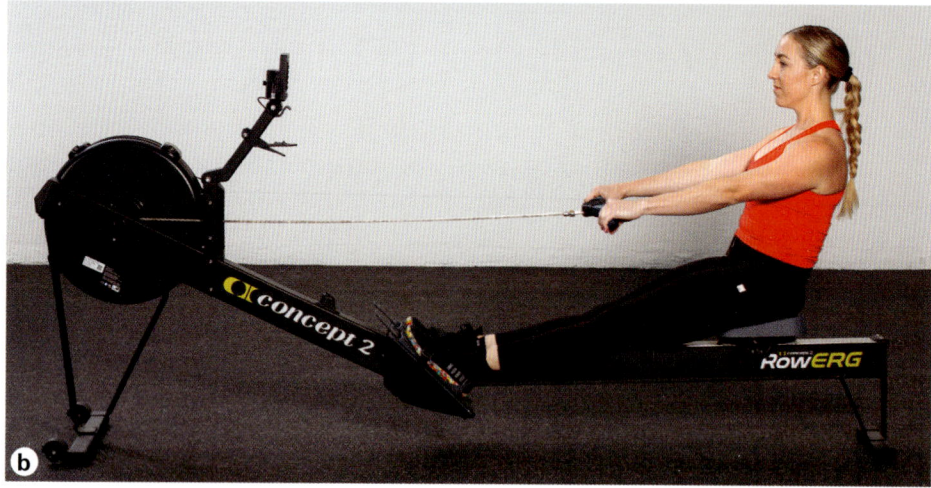

Warm-Up and Cool-Down 97

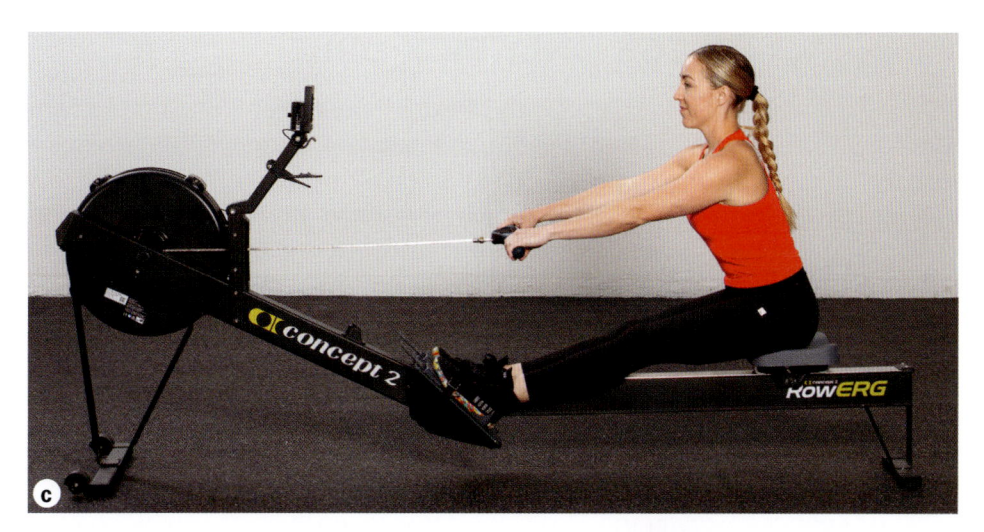

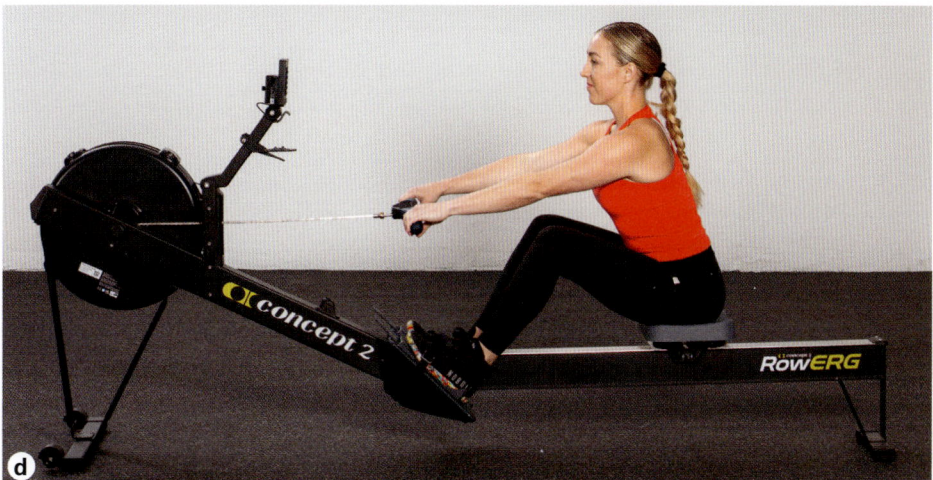

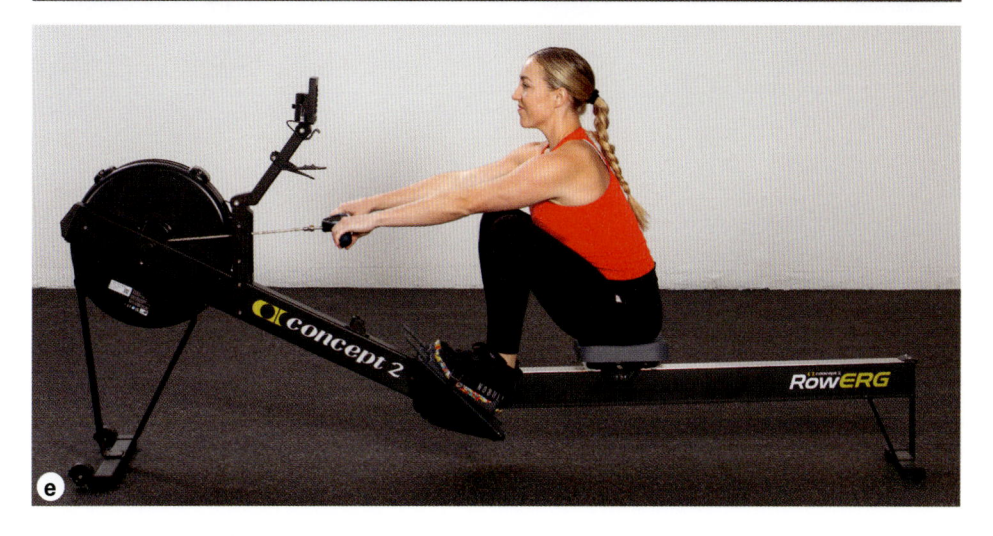

LEGS ONLY PICK DRILL

This drill is very similar to the arms only pick drill; however, this one begins with the legs. It also pieces together the stroke movement by movement. This drill focuses primarily on improving the drive portion of the stroke. Performing this drill well can be very beneficial for adding power and strength to your rowing and core connection. Body positioning and timing are crucial to ensuring you're maximizing the drill's benefits. These drills are only helpful if they are properly performed. Please refer to chapter 4 if you need additional guidance and instructions on either rowing pick drill or proper rowing form.

- Begin in the catch position, extending and contracting only the legs.
- To perform this part of the drill correctly, you must maintain two key performance points.
    - Keep the body in the 11 o'clock (forward) position as you extend the legs *(a)*.
    - Keep a 3:1 ratio to get the most out of the drill: three slow counts in, one strong count back, allowing the handle to get heavy and build resistance.
- Add the upper body swing (hip hinge) so that the legs and body move *(b)*. It's important to hinge before bending your knees on the recovery to activate the legs properly *(c)*. Additionally, to get the most out of this drill, maintain a slow recovery and a strong pushback.
- Add the final arm pull to bring it to a full stroke. This is where you'll get the last 10% of power, and if the drill was performed correctly, you should feel an increase in connection and smooth application of force to the machine *(d)*.

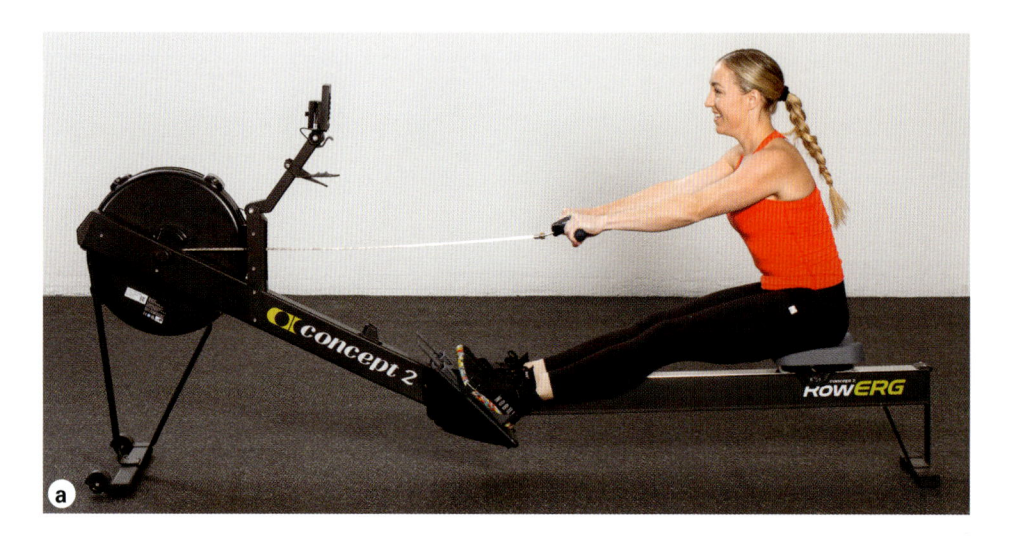

Warm-Up and Cool-Down **99**

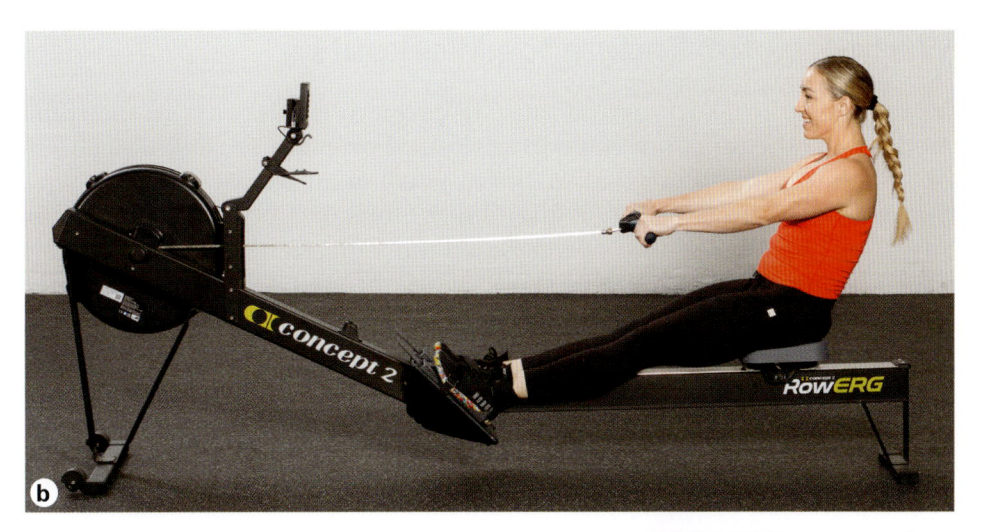

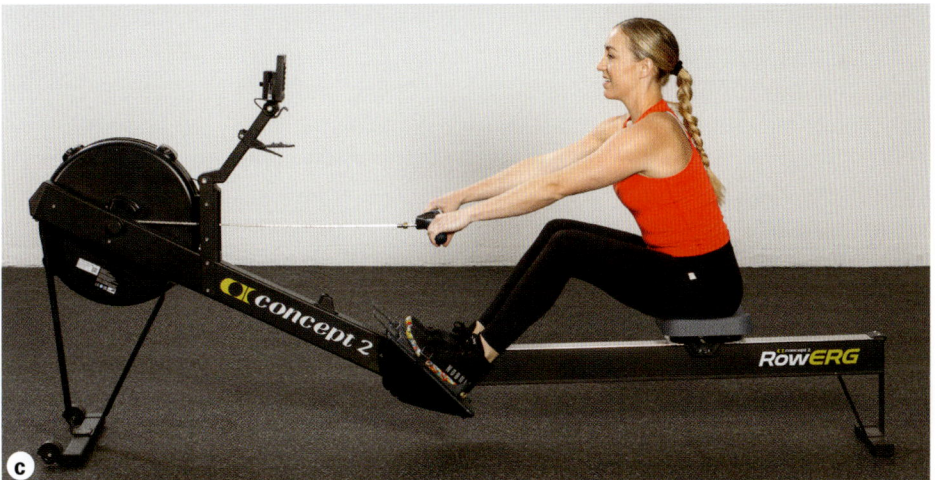

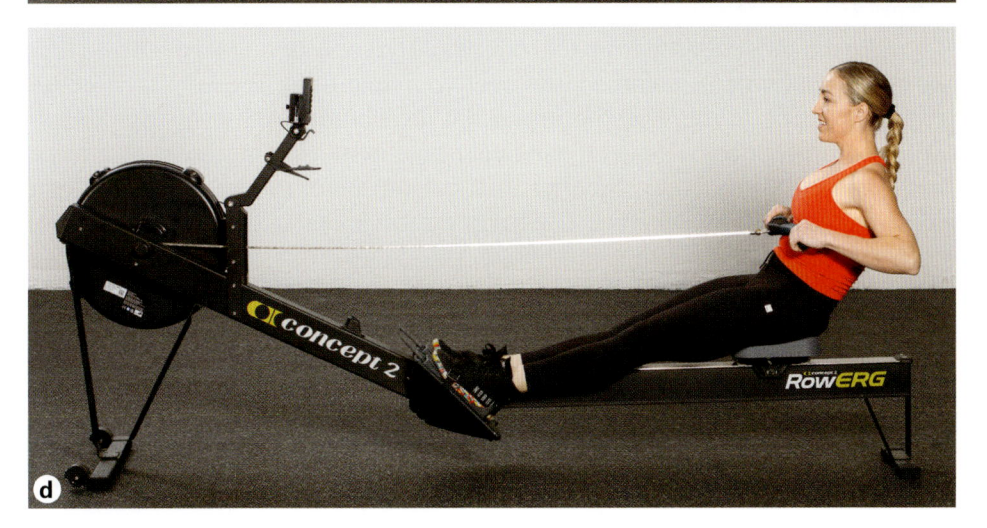

Warm-Ups for Endurance Workouts

It's important to warm up the muscles properly so they are in the right mode to get the most out of your workout. For example, if you're about to do a power-based interval workout, you'll want to warm up in a way that primes your type II, or fast-twitch, muscle fibers, which play a large role in explosive and power-based movements. If you're preparing for an endurance and stamina-based workout, you'll want to prime the slow-twitch muscle fibers, or type I, which are very prevalent in many endurance athletes, like marathon runners. Let's look at some rowing-based warm-ups that would be beneficial if you're preparing your body for an endurance-based workout specifically.

STEADY-STATE ROWING AS A WARM-UP

Steady-state rowing is steadily rowing at a specific cadence at an effort level you can maintain. The suggested intensity is about 50% to 70% effort, like that of a jog. In this warm-up option, we suggest staying under 24 strokes per minute so you can elevate your heart rate slowly while also giving your body the time in the stroke to move with proper form. Many rowers will warm up under 20 strokes per minute, finding a medium-pressure drive with an elongated, controlled recovery. This is a fantastic way to warm up your muscles and create blood and oxygen flow without gassing yourself out for your workout ahead.

STROKE RATE LADDER AS A WARM-UP

Ladders in rowing are often categorized as rate-building pieces to improve stamina, endurance, and control in the stroke. Typically, these are drills in which the stroke rate increases by two strokes for an allotted amount of time, some that go down in rate, and some that go up and come back down.

To gain the most benefit from this drill, you'll not only need to execute control over the stroke rate but also control over your split time. The split time is the time it takes you to row 500 meters, and it recalibrates with every stroke you take. To drop your split, which means your boat is moving faster, you'll need a harder and quicker push on the drive. It is still important to recover slower than you drive back, so you'll want to maintain around a 2:1 ratio, which is two counts on recovery and one count on the drive. The general rule of thumb for stroke rate ladders is that when you go up in strokes per minute, you want to see a slight decrease in split time. As you come back down the ladder and decrease your strokes per minute, you can either allow the split time to increase a few seconds with every stroke rate shift down or, to add additional challenge, aim to maintain the split time as low as possible.

Here are some examples of ladders that are good for a rowing warm-up.

WARM-UP LADDER 1

Look to drop your split time by two to three seconds with each shift up in stroke rate.

- 60 seconds at 18 strokes per minute
- 60 seconds at 20 strokes per minute
- 60 seconds at 22 strokes per minute
- 60 seconds at 24 strokes per minute
- 60 seconds at 26 strokes per minute

WARM-UP LADDER 2

Look to drop your split by four to five seconds with each shift up in stroke rate.

- 2 minutes at 20 strokes per minute
- 90 seconds at 22 strokes per minute
- 60 seconds at 24 strokes per minute
- 30 seconds at 26 strokes per minute

WARM-UP LADDER 3

Look to drop your split by two to three seconds as you increase the rate and maintain a low split as you decrease the stroke rate.

- 90 seconds at 22 strokes per minute
- 60 seconds at 24 strokes per minute
- 30 seconds at 26 strokes per minute
- 60 seconds at 24 strokes per minute
- 90 seconds at 22 strokes per minute

Warm-Ups for Power Workouts

Let's now dive into some warm-ups that would be good if you're preparing your body for a power, HIIT, tabata-style, or really any anaerobic workout. These warm-ups will begin to fire up the fast-twitch, or type II, muscle fibers, allowing your body to prepare for more explosive movements, or in rowing's case, explosive drives or quick catches.

POWER STROKE WARM-UP

Power strokes are very common in rowing, often performed in sets of 10. They are essentially 10 (give or take) powerful strokes done at a specific time. In the sport, many coxswains, or the person steering and coaching the boat, use power 10s to give an extra burst of power and speed to the boat to pull ahead. Oftentimes, these power stroke sets have unique focuses or motivations behind them: "Power 10 for Coach!" In the scenario of using power stroke sets as a warm-up, we can play with the volume of strokes, stroke rate, and unique focus for each set.

One of the main things to consider when doing power strokes for your warm-up is that the intensity needs to shift up or down immediately. This often requires you to row properly. So, the common theme you'll see is that the drills and workouts are most effective with proper rowing form. Below are some power stroke-based warm-ups that work well to prime your fast-twitch muscle fibers. The percentages refer to your maximum effort or perceived exertion.

WARM-UP 1

- Two sets of 10 power strokes at 24 strokes per minute (50%)
- 30-second paddle recovery row between sets
- Two sets of 10 power strokes at 26 strokes per minute (60%)
- 30-second paddle recovery row between sets
- Two sets of 10 power strokes at 28 strokes per minute (70%)
- 30-second paddle recovery row between sets
- Two sets of 10 power strokes at 30 strokes per minute (80%)

WARM-UP 2

Perform a 30-second paddle recovery row between sets. Aim to follow the percentages given based on your perceived exertion.

- 10 power strokes at 22 strokes per minute (50%-60%)
- 15 power strokes at 24 strokes per minute (60%)
- 20 power strokes at 26 strokes per minute (60%-70%)
- 25 power strokes at 28 strokes per minute (70%)
- 30 power strokes at 30 strokes per minute (80%)

The Cool-Down

Cooling down post workout is important to bring control back to your heart and lungs, as well as allow your muscles to recover and begin repairing properly. Depending on your workout, you may consider a few different types of cool-downs. Some cool-downs might include a longer period to allow the heart rate to come down, while others might focus and spend more time on a static stretch.

If you're coming off an anaerobic style, interval, or power-based workout, you might choose to take some time to row steadily or even perform a reverse arms only pick drill. The reverse pick drill simply starts with a light full stroke, then takes away parts of the stroke. You go from full stroke to half stroke, to arms and body only, and finish with just the arms moving out and in. This is a great way to slowly reduce the muscles' work, allowing your heart rate to slowly come down. It also happens to be a great way to reinforce proper movement prior to closing the workout for the day.

Many interval or power-based workouts can create lactic acid buildup. In this case, you may benefit from a light row cool-down to keep the muscles moving in a light effort, slowly flushing the lactic acid. A light, steady row for a few minutes would also work. The general rule of thumb for a cool-down row is to have the goal of regaining control of your breath, so you're back to taking in one inhale and one exhale per stroke. This is a good measure of the heart rate coming down and stabilizing.

> **KEY POINT**
>
> Cooling down post workout is important to bring control back to your heart and lungs, as well as allow your muscles to recover and begin repairing properly.

Once your heart rate has lowered via a light row, consider the following stretches off the rower.

HALF PIGEON STATIC STRETCH

INSTRUCTIONS

- Begin in a plank-like position facing the floor, bring your right knee up toward your chest, and swing your right foot toward the left side of your body *(a)*. Relax into this position, keeping the top of your foot on the ground and your hips squared. Breathe into this position for as much time as you need, then switch sides.
- Keep the arms straight, pressing against the floor with your palms, or go down to your forearms for a deeper stretch *(b)*.

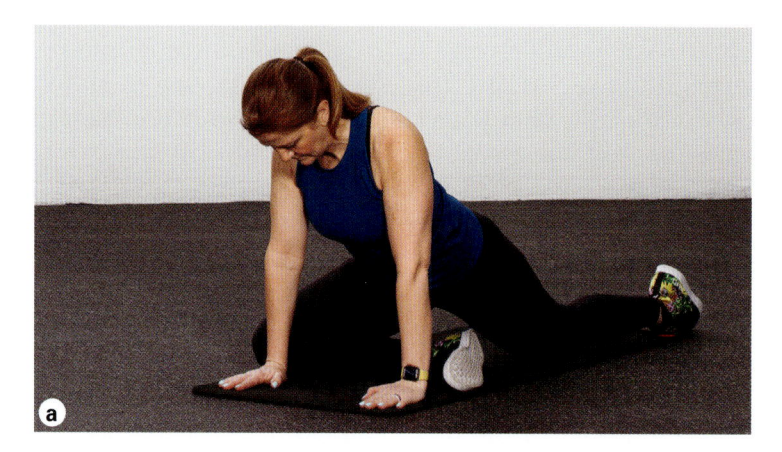

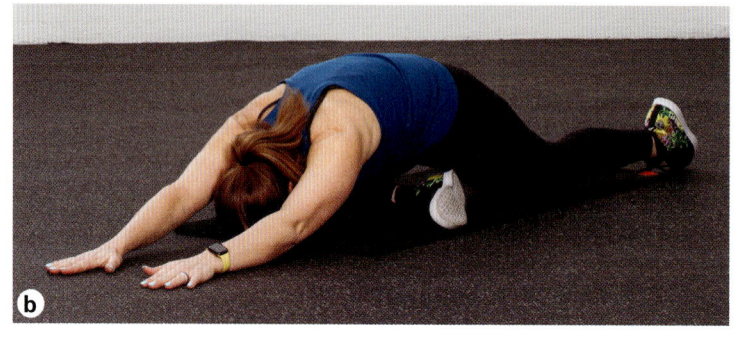

RUNNERS LUNGE + ARM REACH

INSTRUCTIONS

- Place one foot back into a deep lunge and bring your hands to the floor on the inside of your front foot *(a)*.
- Rotate your body toward the front foot as you reach your inside arm toward the sky *(b)*. Hold for about 30 seconds, then switch sides.

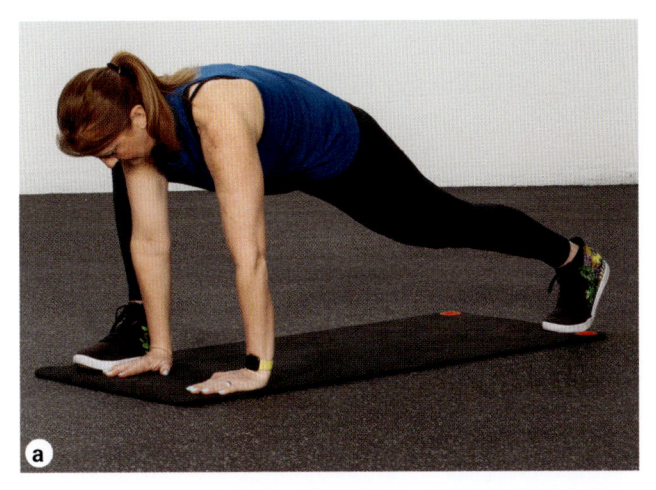

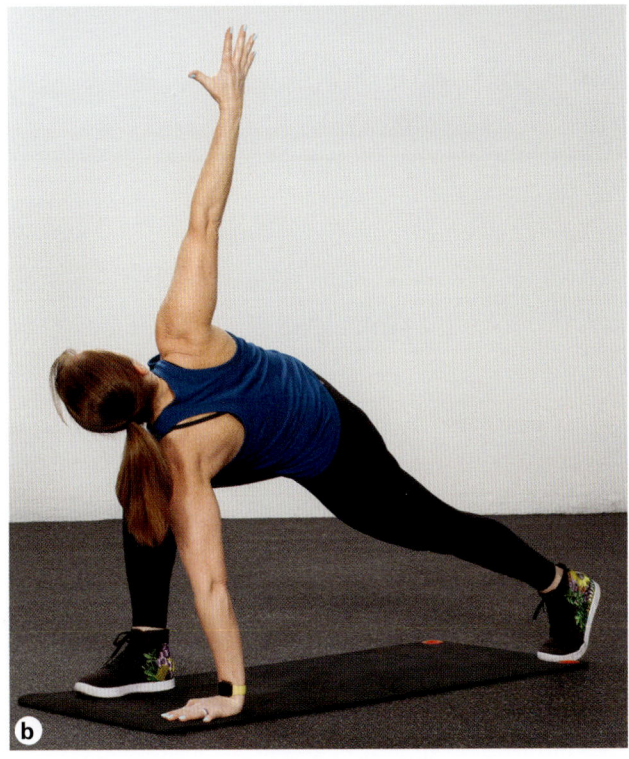

DOWNWARD DOG + HIP SHIFTS AND FOOT PEDALS

INSTRUCTIONS

- Begin in a high plank position, then shift your hips toward the sky. Press your heels into the ground and your head through your arms. Extend both your arms and legs.
- To add the hip shifts, slowly shift your weight to the right, then left *(a)*.
- For the foot pedals, begin to slowly bend one leg and push through the opposite heel for a deeper stretch on that side *(b)*. Alternate the leg that's bending.

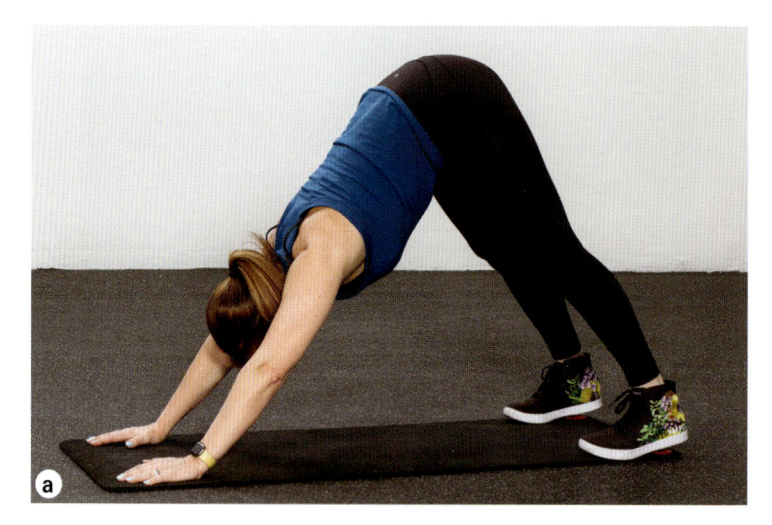

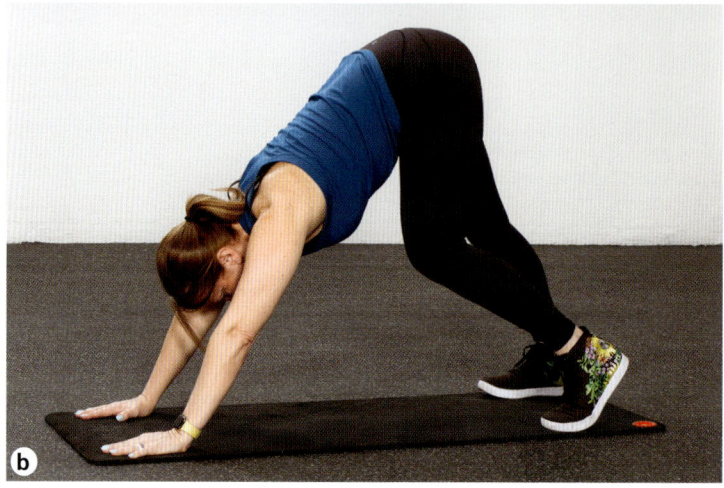

Warm-Up and Cool-Down 107

CAT-COW

See instructions on page 78 earlier in this chapter.

COBRA STRETCH

INSTRUCTIONS

- Bring your body to a prone position (face down), lying on the floor with your hands placed on the ground below your shoulders *(a)*.
- Press against your hands to push your upper body off the ground, straightening your arms if you're able to *(b)*.
- If needed, modify by placing your forearms on the ground rather than your hands, and press up from there.

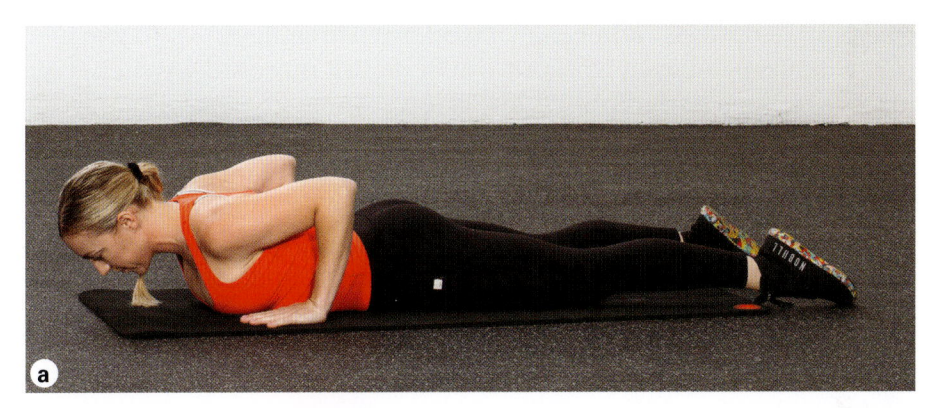

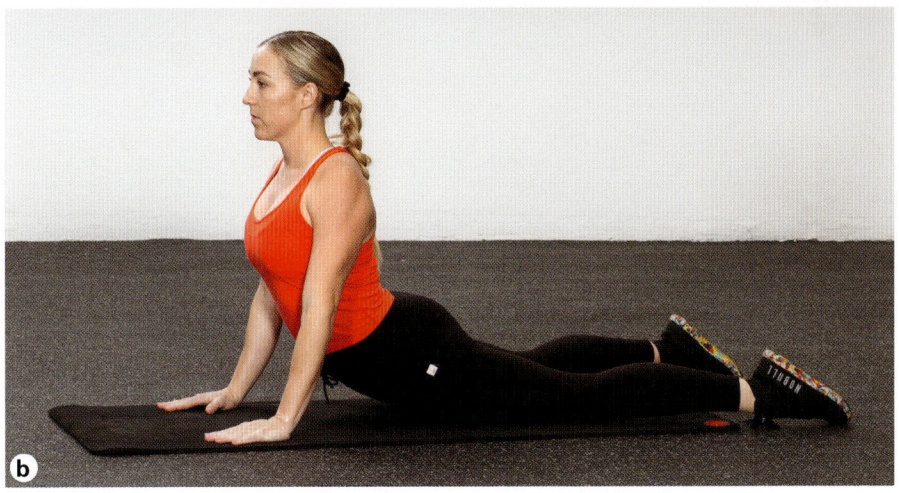

CHILD'S POSE

See instructions on page 80 earlier in this chapter.

    Ultimately, your warm-up should prepare your body for the workout you're about to endure and your cool-down should recover your body from the workout you just performed. We encourage you to note how your body feels during and a few days after a workout to understand if you need to add more to your warm-up or spend more time cooling down and stretching.

    As we dive into endurance and interval-based workouts, consider not only the movement patterns required in the workout but also the type of muscle recruitment required for the workout. For example, an interval workout requires more fast-twitch, type II muscle activation for power, so you might choose to add a bit of speed to your warm-up and one of the power stroke options rather than a ladder if using the rower to warm up. For an endurance-based workout, you'll recruit more slow-twitch, type I muscle fibers, so you might choose a lower-intensity stroke rate ladder.

    Many factors go into choosing the right warm-up or cool-down for the particular workout and for your body. If you're not sure where to start, begin with the warm-ups and cool-downs we've listed here, take the ones you love, and leave the rest. There is no one size fits all for a warm-up, cool-down, or workout. However, having a plan and staying consistent have proven to give results to many people looking to make a change.

7

ENDURANCE WORKOUTS

Endurance training is aerobic, cardiorespiratory exercise that focuses on improving the body's ability to sustain physical activity over a long period. With proper form and an intentional workout plan, rowing can be an excellent form of exercise if endurance is the goal. We know that rowing works the larger muscle groups and recruits most of the body's muscles, resulting in the heart having to work harder to supply blood and oxygen to the body's muscles and organs.

In aerobic workouts, we want the lungs and heart to keep up with the muscles' demands. *Aerobic* means with air. *Anaerobic* means without air. So, when we're approaching an endurance-based workout, we must find an exertion level that allows us to stay consistent over a long period. If we get to the point where our oxygen supply cannot keep up with our exertion level, then we've crossed into the anaerobic training zone, which we'll dive deeper into in the interval training chapter.

We encourage people who are training for general physical fitness and preparedness to train all systems to allow their bodies to be as well rounded as possible. For people who are specifically training for a race or sport that requires strong endurance, we suggest focusing on the aerobic energy system specifically. Additionally, it's important to train not only our cardiorespiratory system but also our muscular system to deliver the best results. As mentioned in chapter 5, there are two types of muscle fibers: type I and type II. Type I muscle fibers are referred to as *slow twitch*, and type II as *fast twitch*. Slow-twitch muscle fibers are typically more abundant in endurance athletes like marathon runners, and fast-twitch fibers are more abundant in power athletes like sprinters.

Before we share three sample endurance workouts, we'll explain a few metrics that are used frequently in rowing. In rowing, we pace ourselves by our 500-meter split time, which is the amount of time you take to row 500 meters with any given stroke. The machine will factor each stroke you take into the split time you see on your monitor. Another important metric is strokes per minute (s/m), which you will see listed in the following workouts. Your strokes per minute are commonly referred to as your stroke rate, which is the number of strokes you're taking each minute, or your cadence. Most rowing machines have both the 500-meter split and stroke rate metrics, although the calibration will vary across different brands of rowers. Therefore, if you're looking to measure and track your training results and progress, you may consider keeping most of your rowing workouts limited to one specific brand of rower. Let's take a peek at three endurance rowing workouts that can result in stronger cardiorespiratory and muscular endurance and stamina.

ENDURANCE WORKOUT #1: 8,500-METER STROKE RATE LADDER

Ladders are a traditional rowing drill in which you increase or decrease the stroke rate at a specified amount of time or distance. This workout will improve your stroke control as you shift rates up and down, as well as challenge your cardiorespiratory system and mental state as your body becomes more and more taxed. The most challenging piece of this workout will be the end of the ladder (as you come down). You will need to recruit more muscles to produce more power because the goal is to maintain the split or speed as you take away strokes per minute. This means fewer strokes and more power. Imagine an outdoor biking drill in which you increased or decreased the gear setting every minute while striving to maintain the same speed. This is essentially the same idea. It requires a lot of control, focus, and stamina! Most rowing is performed at a 1:2 timing ratio from drive to recovery. During this ladder drill, you'll find the most success by adjusting your timing slightly as you go up in stroke rate and come back down. As you go up in stroke rate, you'll want to maintain the drive speed and quicken the recovery, while still ensuring the drive is slightly quicker than the recovery. In order to maintain your split time low on the way down the ladder, you'll need to lengthen through the recovery and speed up the drive. This is the tricky part!

When reading the workout, you'll see the number of meters to row, the desired strokes per minute (s/m), and 500-meter split guidance. Perform the first 1,000 meters at a moderate intensity, then use the split from that piece to determine your split goals for the remainder of the workout. When the workout says *–1 second off split*, aim to drop your split by 1 second from the previous piece. When you're coming back down the stroke rate ladder, your goal is to maintain the split exactly where you had it on the 500 meters at 28 strokes per minute. It is important not to start this workout with too much intensity, as you will risk burning out too quickly. The total workout is 8,500 meters, which will take most people anywhere from 35 to 60 minutes, so be sure to begin at a pace that allows you to pick up intensity and speed throughout the time; be patient and focus on consistency and control.

- 1,000 meters at 18 s/m
- 900 meters at 20 s/m (*–1 second off split*)
- 800 meters at 22 s/m (*–1 second off split*)
- 700 meters at 24 s/m (*–1 second off split*)
- 600 meters at 26 s/m (*–1 second off split*)
- 500 meters at 28 s/m (*–1 second off split*)

- 600 meters at 26 s/m (aim to maintain split)
- 700 meters at 24 s/m (aim to maintain split)
- 800 meters at 22 s/m (aim to maintain split)
- 900 meters at 20 s/m (aim to maintain split)
- 1,000 meters at 18 s/m (aim to maintain split)

If you want to explore ladders but this workout seems too daunting to begin with, we've included two additional workouts here that can be great starting points. For both drills, you'll want to adopt a similar pacing strategy as this first drill, dropping your split as you go up in stroke rate and aiming to maintain the low split as you come back down in stroke rate.

11-MINUTE LADDER DRILL

- 60 seconds at 20 s/m
- 60 seconds at 22 s/m (*–1 second off split*)
- 60 seconds at 24 s/m (*–1 second off split*)
- 60 seconds at 26 s/m (*–1 second off split*)
- 60 seconds at 28 s/m (*–1 second off split*)
- 60 seconds at 30 s/m (*–1 second off split*)
- 60 seconds at 28 s/m (aim to maintain split)
- 60 seconds at 26 s/m (aim to maintain split)
- 60 seconds at 24 s/m (aim to maintain split)
- 60 seconds at 22 s/m (aim to maintain split)
- 60 seconds at 20 s/m (aim to maintain split)

9.5-MINUTE LADDER DRILL

- 2 minutes at 22 s/m
- 90 seconds at 24 s/m (*–1 second off split*)
- 60 seconds at 26 s/m (*–1 second off split*)
- 30 seconds at 28 s/m (*–1 second off split*)
- 60 seconds at 26 s/m (aim to maintain split)
- 90 seconds at 24 s/m (aim to maintain split)
- 2 minutes at 22 s/m (aim to maintain split)

ENDURANCE WORKOUT #2: STEADY REPEAT

Steady rowing is very similar to running in the sense that it's almost as much of a mental game as a physical one. It's important to find consistency in your rowing stroke so you can control your exertion. Efficiency is key here. The drive portion of the stroke moves the boat, so the idea is to relax as much as possible on the recovery and make the most out of the drive with proper muscular connection and stroke timing. Just like people find their zone when running, we rowers find our groove as we endure these longer rows. Music helps!

- Steady row for 5,000 meters (5K).
  - Choose a rate between 22 and 24 s/m and stick with it.
  - Aim to drop your split time by 1 second for each 1,000 meters you accumulate.
- Rest for 5 minutes.
- Steady row for 5,000 meters.
  - Choose the same stroke rate (s/m) as the previous piece.
  - Aim to match or drop your split from the previous round (see figure 7.1).

As mentioned in chapter 5, music can be a game changer for your mental focus during a workout or training session. When aiming to maintain a specific stroke rate for a long time, it can be helpful to find music at that specific rate. Once you have selected your stroke rate, multiply it by 4 and find music that has the same beats per minute. This additional step may take a bit of extra time to pull together before your workout, but it will pay off!

KEY POINT

Find music that has a similar cadence to your rowing, so each stroke is consistent.

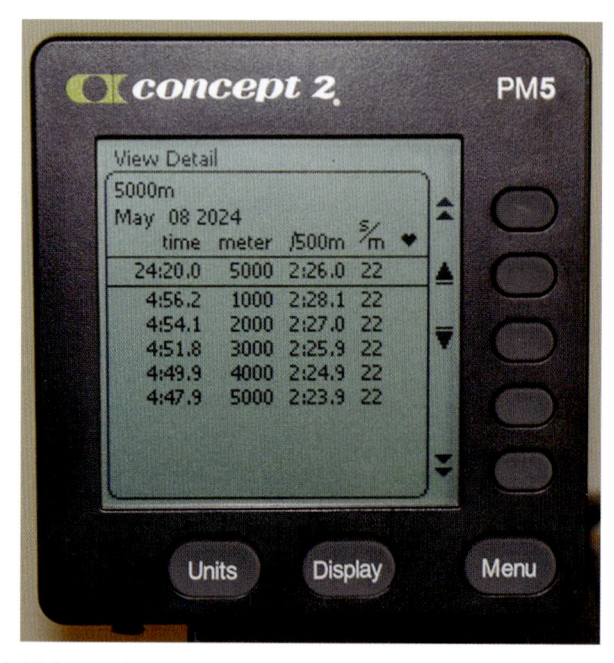

FIGURE 7.1 Hold the stroke rate, and aim to drop the split time by 1 second every 1,000 meters.

Courtesy of Caley Crawford

ENDURANCE WORKOUT #3: DESCENDING 6,000-METER ROW

This workout essentially breaks down a 6-kilometer row into pieces. It requires more muscle recruitment as you reduce the stroke rate. Why is that? We want you to maintain your split the entire time, so you'll need to put more force into each stroke. When we take fewer strokes per minute, more effort is required to keep the boat moving at the same pace, or speed. To complete this workout with precision, you must have complete control over the stroke and the recovery.

- 3,000 meters at 26 s/m
- 2,000 meters at 22 s/m (aim to maintain split)
- 1,000 meters at 18 s/m (aim to maintain split)

If you find it difficult to maintain the split, your conditioning might need improvement, in which case it will get better with time and workouts! The lack of consistency could also be due to a lack of control and consistency in your stroke form. If this is the case, we encourage you to go back and do some of the stroke-improvement drills from chapter 4.

If you find yourself struggling to understand how to lower the stroke rate while still maintaining speed, do the exercise on the next page for practice before approaching the full 6,000-meter workout. It's a quick exercise, so it takes the conditioning variable out of the equation, which should allow you to focus solely on control.

- 300 meters at 26 s/m
- 200 meters at 22 s/m (aim to maintain split)
- 100 meters at 18 s/m (aim to maintain split)

The goal is to maintain your split throughout. On the shifts down in stroke rate, be sure to add a stronger drive through the legs and a longer recovery because you'll have to add more power per stroke in order to maintain your split.

When you make the shift down in stroke rate, the goal is to have enough control that you can adjust the stroke rate and lengthen the recovery in one stroke. The drive must increase in strength and quickness, while the recovery must lengthen and slow down immediately. Keep trying this exercise until you can successfully maintain a low split throughout the shift. Bonus points if you can drop your split time even more on the lower stroke rate! If you are still struggling after a few attempts, it's likely due to the sequence and timing of your recovery. The body over pause drill on page 43 can be a great exercise for improving the recovery sequence in your stroke.

Endurance workouts are simple; however, they require control, consistency, and efficiency in the rowing movement in order to maximize effectiveness. The workouts get easier over time as you work to build that consistency, as well as your mental focus and cardiorespiratory fitness.

8

INTERVAL WORKOUTS

Interval training enhances your cardiorespiratory fitness and improves heart rate variability by alternating higher intensity bursts of energy with lower intensity recovery periods. While intervals don't always have to be high intensity, interval training is typically higher intensity, focused on training the anaerobic energy system, which provides specific results and benefits to the body. One of the heart rate identifiers for improvement in your training is how quickly your heart recovers to a manageable rate. Over time, with training, you should see your heart recover a lot faster. If you looked at the heart rate graph of a trained and conditioned athlete doing interval training, you might see something like the graph in figure 8.1: strong peaks and valleys.

On the other hand, for someone who's deconditioned or just getting started on their interval training journey, you might see something like the image in figure 8.2, with a longer recovery time and less recovery because the heart rate doesn't dip as low.

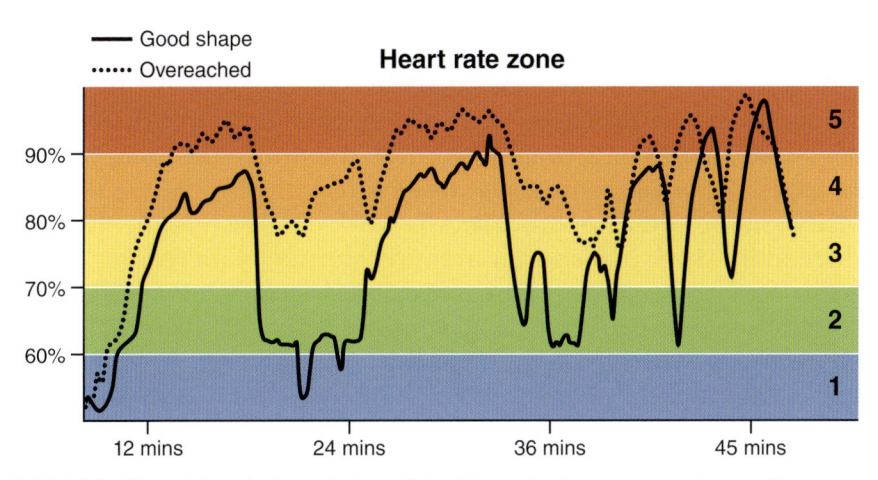

FIGURE 8.1 The athlete in "good shape" is able to do the same workout without exerting the heart as much in the beginning and shows stronger heart rate recovery during the rest periods of the intervals.

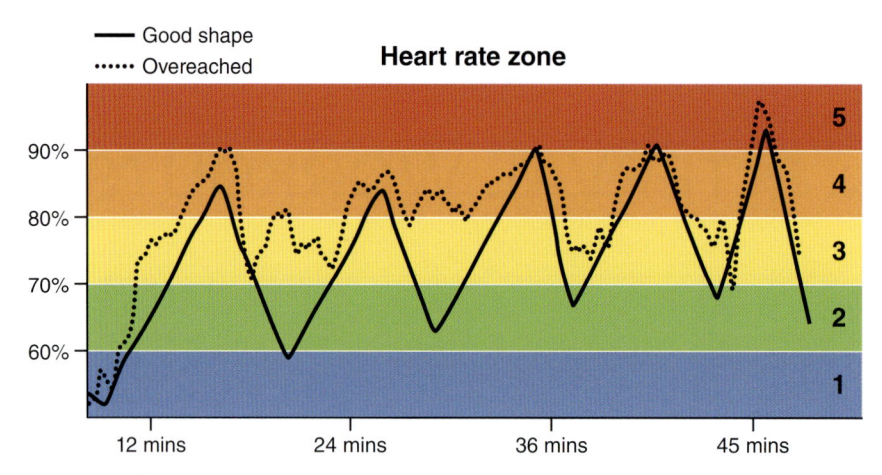

FIGURE 8.2 This diagram shows the heart rate map during an interval workout, comparing someone who's less conditioned to someone who's more conditioned. Notice that the person who is in "good shape" has strong recovery during the less intense moments of the workout.

Most high-intensity interval training will put you in an anaerobic cardiorespiratory zone. *Anaerobic* means without air. Essentially, this means your body and muscles are working so hard that your blood flow and oxygen intake cannot keep up. Some people may call it *redlining* or *maxing out* your cardiorespiratory system. The rower is often a first choice for interval training because it works so many muscles at once. When you work larger muscle groups and recruit more muscles in a specific exercise, your heart must work harder. So, it allows you to find that anaerobic zone quickly on a machine like the rower.

Although it is possible to find intensity at lower stroke rates, high-intensity interval training on the rowing machine typically occurs at higher stroke rates. Once you learn how to maximize the force you apply to the machine, bringing up your stroke rate will allow you to maximize intensity and power. After all, power is work divided by time. If you can produce more work in a shorter amount of time by increasing the rate, you will create more power (more strokes in less time). Higher rates will also allow you to find an anaerobic zone because you will have a quicker stroke recovery, which will not allow you to catch your breath between each stroke. Eventually, your work will max out your oxygen supply.

Let's look at some ways to perform interval training using the rowing machine. Notice that many of the following workout examples are short. The beauty of interval training is that you can do a lot of work in a very short amount of time. Whether you're looking to do only intervals for your workout or just need a quick cardio blast at the end of a workout, these options are for you! As you put these workouts into practice, be sure to review chapter 6 and warm up and cool down properly. Due to the high intensity and fast-twitch muscle activation these workouts require, your performance in the workout itself will improve, as will your body's ability to recover.

Due to the short duration (20 seconds or 10 strokes) of many of these interval workouts, we encourage using a sprint start to maximize the time spent on the work portion of the workout. What is a sprint start? It is a way that we can get the flywheel (or water) moving quickly in a short amount of time. It essentially allows us to maximize the work by aggressively and efficiently putting force into the machine that results in the flywheel momentum building quickly.

Let's look at a sprint start example (figure 8.3): Half stroke, half stroke, three-fourths stroke, full stroke.

There are a few different versions of a sprint start depending on where you row and what feels right, but the example above is the one that many people use in their training.

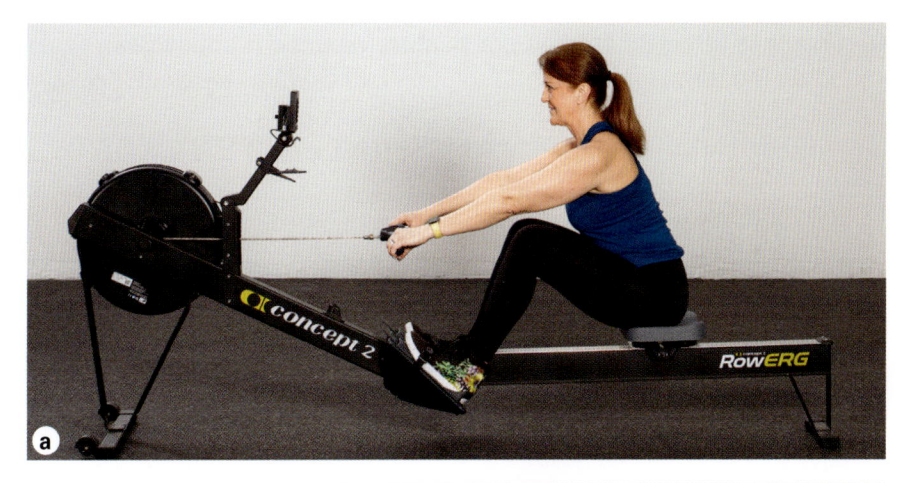

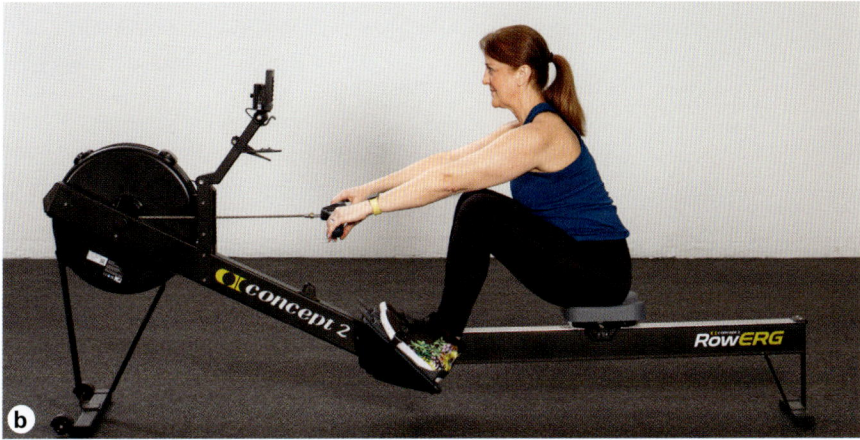

FIGURE 8.3 *(a)* Half stroke and *(b)* three-fourths stroke.

1:1 WORK-TO-REST RATIO

10 rounds, one-minute max-effort row, one-minute full rest

TABATA BLAST: 2:1 WORK-TO-REST RATIO

Eight rounds, 20-seconds max effort, 10-seconds full recovery

The goal for both workouts is to hit the same split for each round of sprints. The stroke rate can be as high as you want, as long as you maintain proper form. The suggested stroke rate range is 28 to 36 strokes per minute.

15-MINUTE POWER STROKE EMOM (EVERY MINUTE ON THE MINUTE)

10 strokes max effort, rest for the seconds remaining

The goal is to produce the same wattage for each set of 10 strokes. The stroke rate can be as high as you want, as long as you maintain proper form. The suggested range is 28 to 36 strokes per minute. Wattage produced can typically be found on most rowing machine monitors by adjusting the units displayed.

10 MINUTES OF VANISHING INTERVALS

- 2-minute max row
- 2-minute rest
- 90-second max row
- 90-second rest
- 60-second max row
- 60-second rest
- 30-second max row
- 30-second rest

You may have noticed that these suggested workouts have short training intervals that range from 4 to 20 minutes. Due to rowing's full-body nature, your body is going to find your anaerobic threshold quickly, making your workouts incredibly efficient. Imagine doing a strength workout and then ending with a series of rowing intervals to blast out all the muscles and the cardiorespiratory system. Whether you have only 4 minutes or more than 20, there are effective options for you. Very few cardiorespiratory workouts that are also full body and low impact allow you to find an anaerobic energy zone in such a short amount of time.

PART IV

CUSTOMIZE YOUR PROGRAM

9

OFF-THE-ROWER STRENGTH TRAINING FOR ON-THE-ROWER PERFORMANCE

Take your training OFF the rower to find power ON the rower! Rowing is a technical sport that requires a high level of proprioception to do well. Building muscle and body awareness off the rower will give you gains over time on the rower. Rowing at a higher intensity requires a large oxygen uptake. Strength and power training will increase strength, mobility, and flexibility, giving you the overall push you need to reach those lower splits.

> ### KEY POINT
> Building muscle and body awareness off the rower will give you gains over time on the rower.

Remember, prior to starting any strength training program, get approval from your physician. It is also recommended that you find a qualified personal trainer to assist you with performing these exercises correctly if you're new to strength training.

Off-the-rower training can be broken into two categories:

1. Movements that mimic the rowing stroke (complementary movements)
2. Movements that support the rowing stroke (supplemental movements)

Both are necessary for finding balance when strengthening all the muscles used in rowing. Rowers who don't incorporate strength training into their program are likely to develop muscular imbalances, which can greatly diminish performance.

Complementary Movements

Complementary movements are simple to identify and provide specificity to off-the-rower training. Complementary movements focus on building muscles that support the rowing stroke and muscles necessary for the stroke. We'll focus on the glutei (glutes), the hamstrings, the quadriceps (quads), the core, and the latissimus dorsi (lats).

> **KEY POINT**
>
> Complementary movements focus on building muscles that support the rowing stroke and muscles necessary for the stroke.

To determine your ideal weight, choose a weight that allows you to do the first set of 10 repetitions with moderate difficulty (Hunter et al. 2015). The last few reps should be difficult, but not so difficult that you're straining through the movement. If that happens, lighten the weight for the next set. Beginners should start with 3 sets of 8 to 12 reps. Choose the weight that allows you to finish all the sets with good form. If you want to increase strength, your goal should be fewer repetitions with a heavier weight. Ensure that you have established a strong baseline before picking up heavier weights.

Gluteus

The gluteus muscles are easily the strongest muscles in the body. They consist of three muscles: the gluteus maximus, gluteus medius, and gluteus minimus. These three muscles control the hip in extension, hyperextension, abduction, and external rotation. The glutes also play a huge role in hip stabilization. For that reason, you want to ensure that you're giving attention to all three muscles. Two exercises to develop the glutes follow.

BARBELL HIP THRUST

INSTRUCTIONS

- Set up a loaded barbell (you can also use dumbbells) and a weight bench in a place where it won't move.
- Sit on the ground next to the long side of the bench with your legs straight and your back pressed against the bench. Place the barbell directly over your hips.
- Bend your knees, pulling your feet closer to your glutes, so your shins are vertical and your feet flat *(a)*. You can rest your hands on the barbell.
- Brace your core and thrust your hips up toward the sky *(b)*. At the same time, squeeze your glutes and press your feet into the ground.
- Slowly return to the starting position and repeat for the desired number of repetitions.

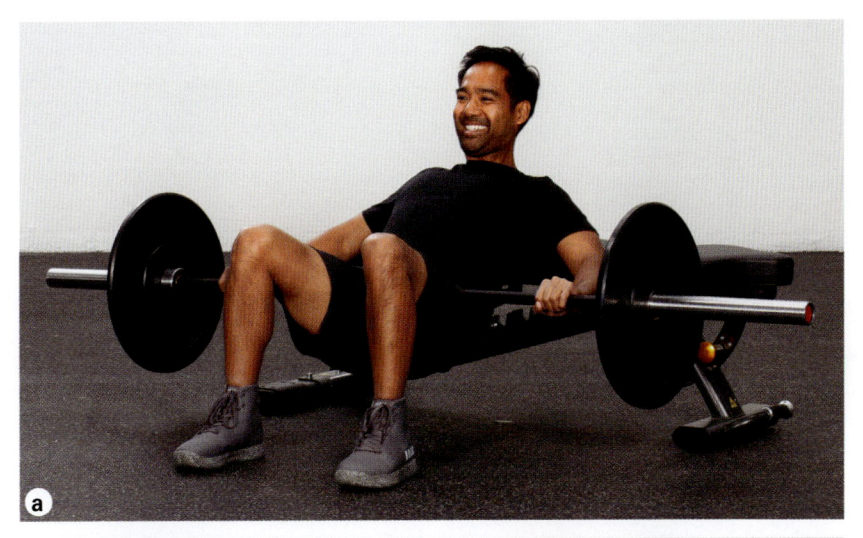

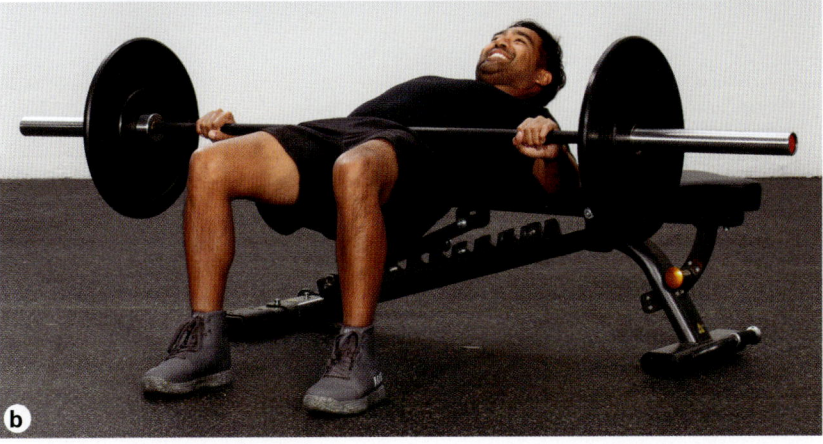

SPLIT SQUAT

INSTRUCTIONS

- Stand with your feet about shoulder-width apart. Step back about 12 to 18 inches with one foot; your back heel should be lifted so you're on the ball of your foot *(a)*. Your back knee should be soft, with most of your weight on your front leg.
- Brace your core.
- Maintaining a tall torso, lower your back knee toward the floor *(b)*. The front knee will bend as a result. Keep your weight in your front foot. At the bottom of the movement, both legs should be at 90-degree angles.
- Drive through your front foot to return to a standing position. Repeat for the desired number of repetitions.

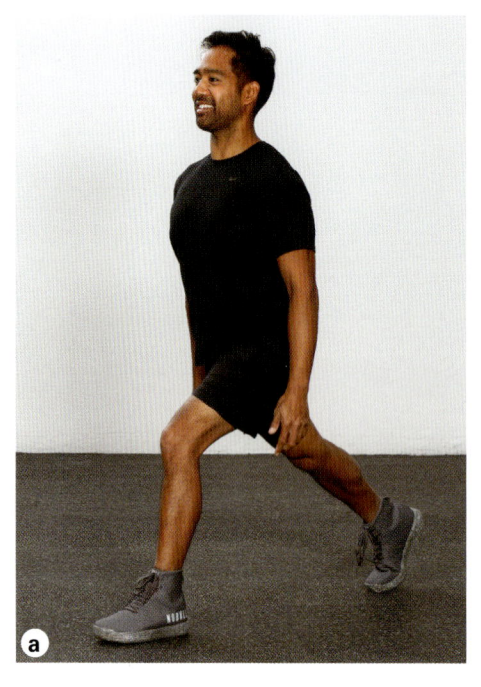

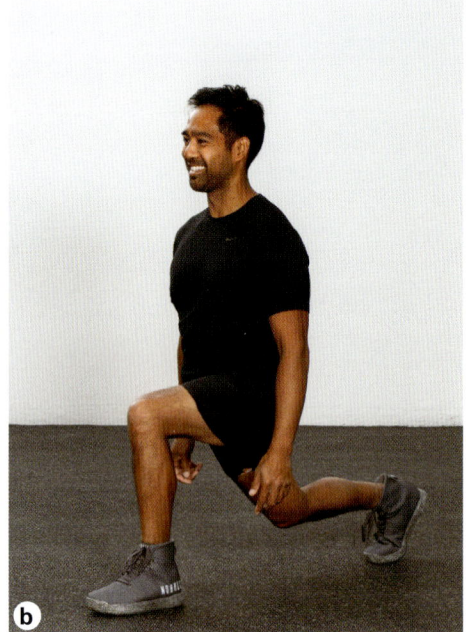

Hamstrings

The hamstrings are another group of three muscles (biceps femoris, semimembranosus, and semitendinosus). The hamstrings are responsible for hip extension and knee flexion. In the rowing stroke, the hamstrings help to flex the knees to bring you back to the front of the stroke. In the very first part of the drive, they are active until the knees extend. It is critical to have hamstrings that are not only strong but flexible. With that in mind, we are going to focus on two movements, one for strength and one for flexibility.

ROMANIAN DEADLIFT (STRENGTH)

INSTRUCTIONS

- Stand tall with your feet hip-distance apart and a soft bend in your knees. Grip the barbell or dumbbells overhand, about shoulder-width apart.
- Your arms should hang directly down from your shoulder joints. Brace your lats and core *(a)*.
- Hinge at the hips and slowly begin to lower the weight toward the floor. Lead backward with your hips, keeping the weight in contact with your legs and your back lengthened and active. Lower only as far as your hamstrings allow while maintaining a neutral spine *(b)*.
- Squeeze the glutes and press the hips forward as you return to standing. Repeat for the desired number of repetitions.

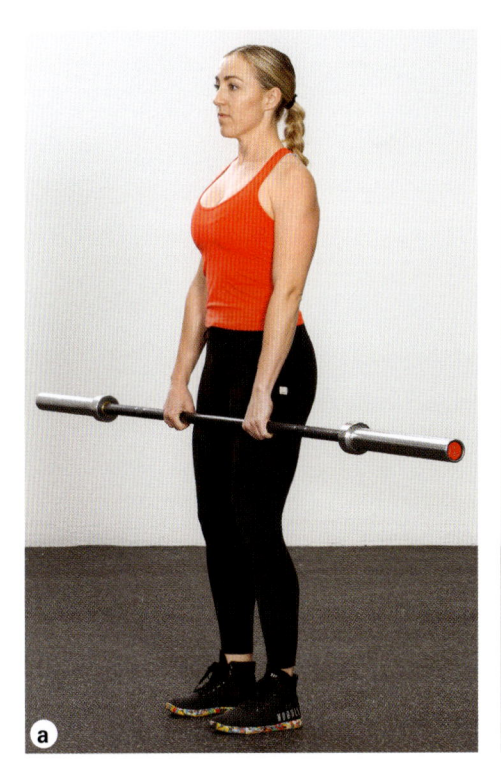

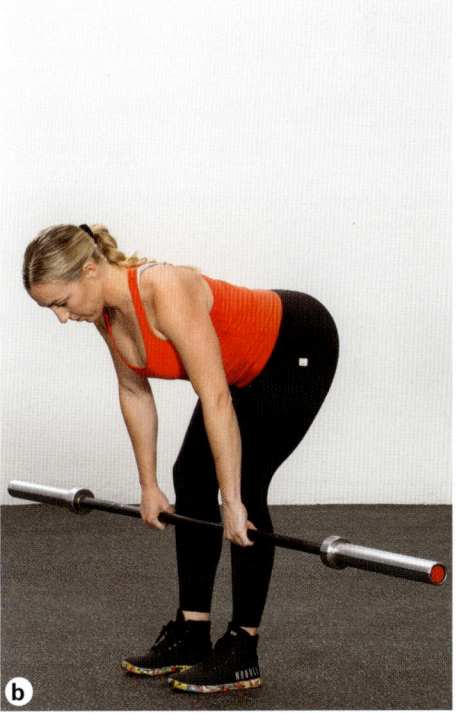

TOWEL HAMSTRINGS STRETCH (FLEXIBILITY)

INSTRUCTIONS

- Sit on the floor with your legs extended in front of you.
- Loop a long towel, belt, or strap around the ball of one foot and hold the ends of the towel or strap in either hand *(a)*. The opposite leg should remain flat on the floor, outstretched and actively pressing into the floor.
- While keeping your chest lifted, shoulders back, and spine long, slowly lift the belted leg until you feel a stretch in your hamstrings *(b)*. Hold for 30 seconds and relax.
- Repeat three to five times before switching legs.

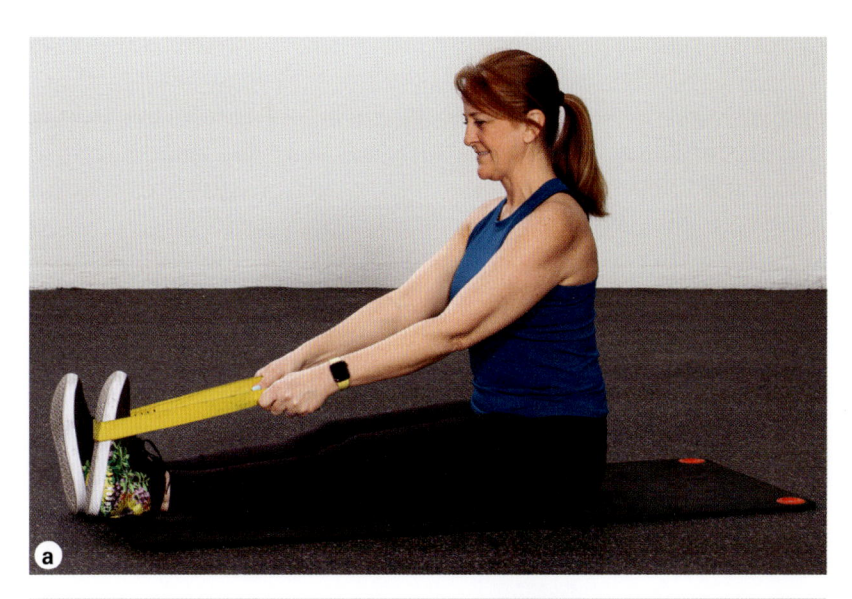

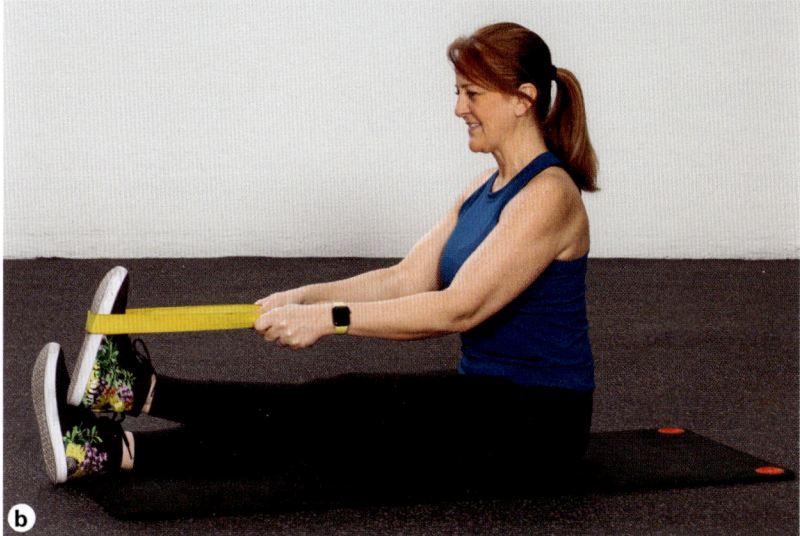

Quadriceps

The quadriceps consist of four muscles: the rectus femoris, vastus lateralis, vastus medialis, and vastus intermedius. The quads' main job is hip flexion and knee extension. Vastus medialis, vastus intermedius, and vastus lateralis also stabilize the patella.

Strong quads are a must for a healthy stroke! The quads are one of the primary movers in the drive, helping to propel you from the front to the back of the machine. To generate force and power, push against the foot stretcher as though you are jumping away from the front of the machine. Powerful quads allow for a powerful drive.

We're going to focus on two explosive movements that will help build this power. These are plyometric movements. This means that your feet will leave the ground. A low-impact version is available by keeping your feet planted, lowering slowly, and exploding up to standing.

JUMP SQUAT

INSTRUCTIONS

- Stand with your feet shoulder-width apart and your knees slightly bent. Your arms will be hanging by your sides.
- Engage your core and bend your knees to drop to a full squat position. As you drop down, extend your arms out in front of your body at chest height *(a)*.
- Engage through your quads, glutes, and hamstrings to propel your body up and off the floor, swinging your arms down and back to allow you to activate through the core. Fully extend your hips and knees at the top of the movement *(b)*.
- Land softly and repeat for the desired number of repetitions.

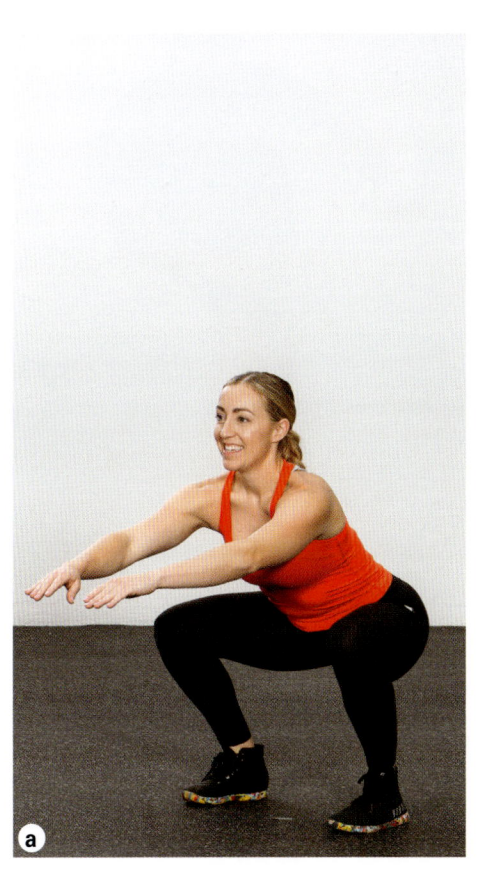

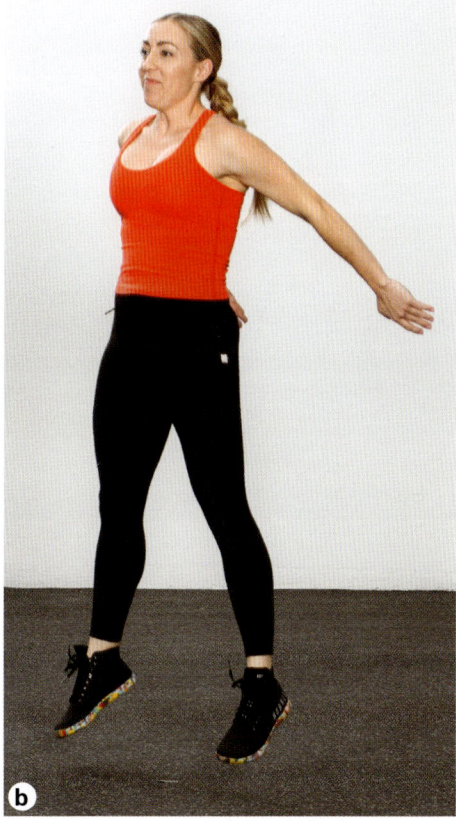

SKATER JUMP

INSTRUCTIONS

- Stand with your feet together and knees slightly bent, with your arms resting at your sides.
- Brace your core and shift your weight to the left leg.
- Push off the left leg to jump to the right, bringing your left foot behind you and your left arm in front of your chest in a curtsy lunge position *(a-b)*.
- Repeat on the other side, moving back and forth at a brisk pace, for the desired number of repetitions.

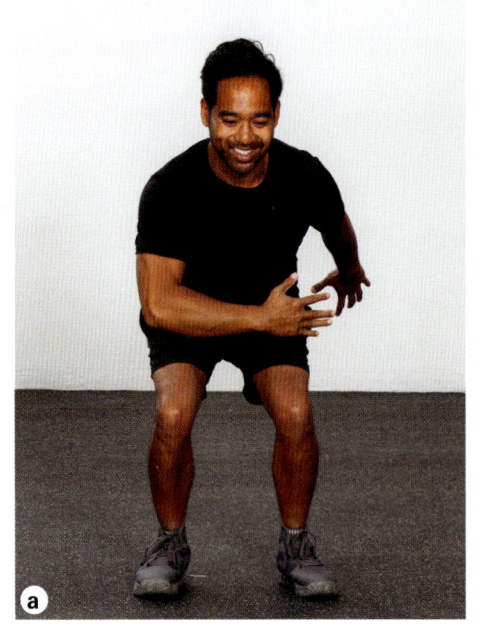

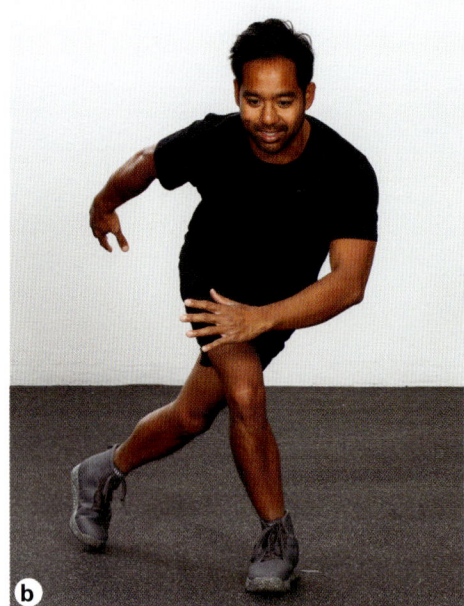

Core

The core is the center of the body and is the point from which all movement originates. The core includes your hips and pelvis, as well as the muscles in the back and front of the torso. On the rower, your core is active 100% of the time. Your core is the connector between your lower body and the handle, and an efficient transfer of power can only happen if your core remains active.

Core movements fall into two categories: core strength and core stabilization. Core strength is the ability to produce force throughout a given movement (e.g., crunches). Stability refers to the ability to resist unwanted movement (e.g., planks). We'll focus here on both, because both are necessary for the rowing stroke.

SUITCASE MARCH (STABILIZATION)

INSTRUCTIONS

- Stand with your feet hip-distance apart, arms hanging by your sides. Hold a dumbbell in your right hand. You can use your left arm extended out for balance if needed.
- Brace your core, keep your chest up and your shoulders and hips square.
- March in place or walk for 30 to 60 seconds.
- Switch the dumbbell to the left hand and repeat.

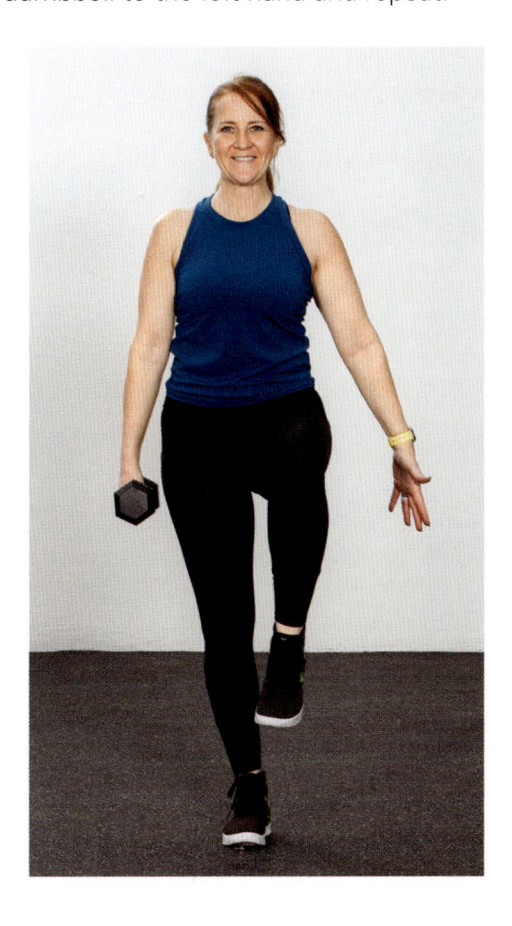

MEDICINE BALL SLAMS (STRENGTH)

INSTRUCTIONS

- Stand with your feet hip-distance apart and knees slightly bent, holding a medicine ball in your hands.
- Extend your arms overhead and brace your core *(a)*.
- Hinge forward at the hips and use your core muscles to slam the ball against the floor in front of you, bending your knees and lowering your hips into a squat *(b)*. Let your arms follow through and return to standing, catching the ball as it bounces up or reaching down while bending the knees further to pick up the ball from the floor.
- Repeat for the desired number of repetitions.

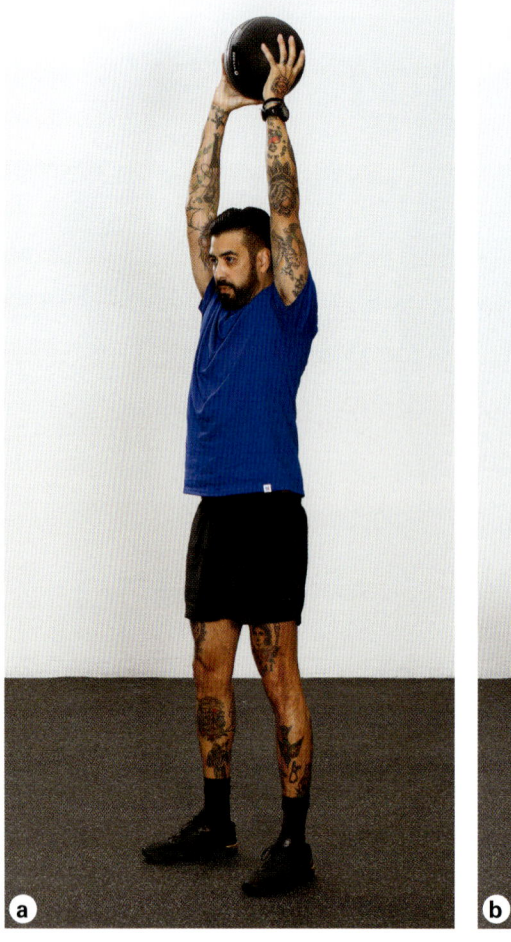

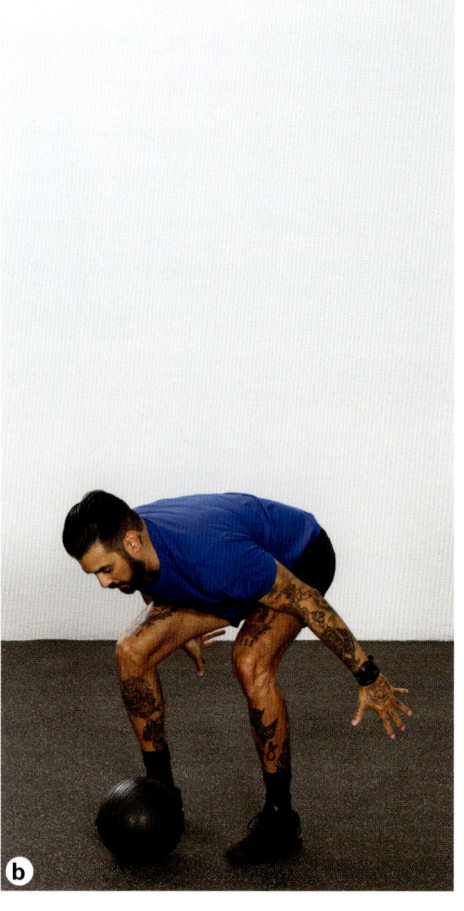

TIP If you use a medicine ball that bounces, be very careful that the ball doesn't hit you in the face after you slam it to the floor. It's best to use a medicine ball specifically designed for slamming.

Latissimus Dorsi

The latissimus dorsi are the large fan-shaped muscles on your back. They're attached to your ribs, spine, upper arms, and scapula. They're a major pulling muscle in the upper body and are responsible for internal rotation, adduction, and extension of the arms. The lats help in the rowing stroke by stabilizing on the drive and pulling the handle toward the chest at the finish. They also help with control at the beginning of the recovery sequence as you release your arms forward. We've selected two basic but effective movements to help build strength in the lats.

BENT-OVER ROW

INSTRUCTIONS

- Stand with your feet hip-distance apart, holding a dumbbell in each hand.
- Keep your spine straight, brace your core, and hinge forward at the hips. Keep a soft bend in your knees and allow your arms to hang directly below your shoulders *(a)*.
- Bend your elbows and slowly draw the head of the dumbbells back toward your hips *(b)*.
- Pause and then slowly lower the weights to the starting position.
- Repeat for the desired number of repetitions.

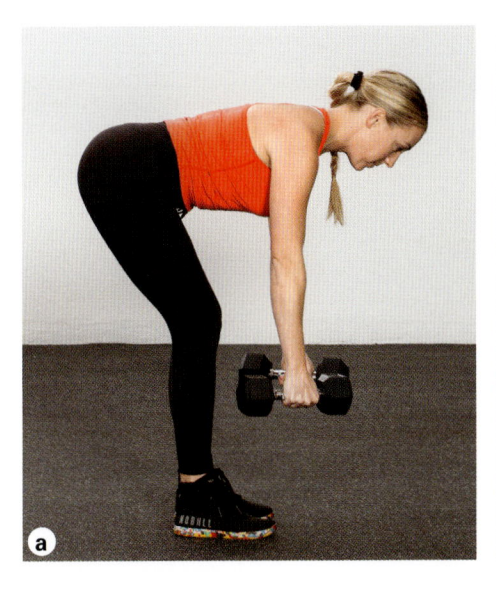

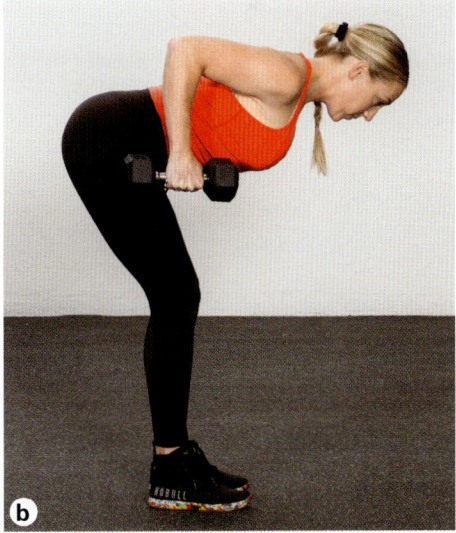

DUMBBELL PULLOVER

INSTRUCTIONS

- Lie flat on a bench or on the floor, holding the head of one dumbbell with both hands.
- With the dumbbell in your hands, extend your arms up toward the ceiling *(a)*.
- Keeping your feet planted and core braced, extend the dumbbell overhead, maintaining a slight bend in the elbows *(b)*. Slowly and with control, bring the dumbbell back to its starting position.
- Repeat for the desired number of repetitions.

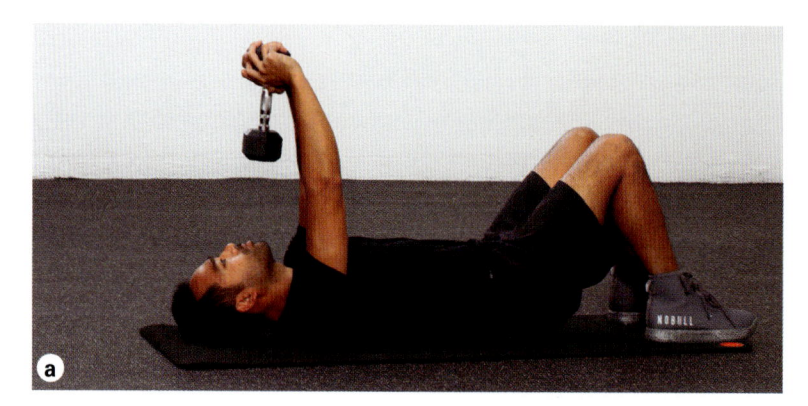

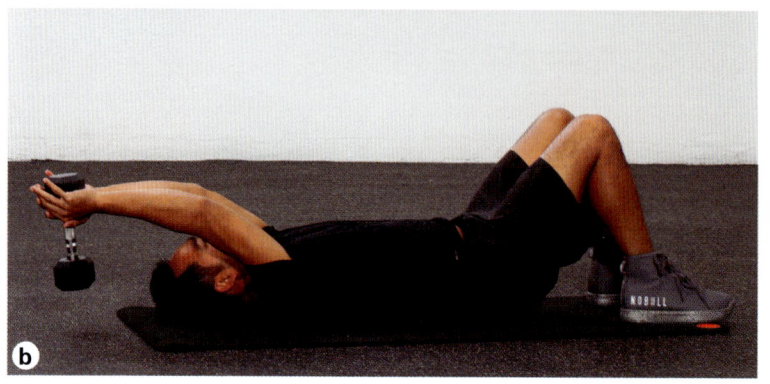

Supplemental Movements

Supplemental movements focus on building the muscles that rowing does not address: mainly the upper body pressing muscles, including the chest, shoulders, and triceps, and the spinal erector muscles, including the erector spinae and the transversospinalis muscle group. This type of training is necessary for muscular balance and will provide a good foundation for injury prevention.

> **KEY POINT**
>
> Supplemental movements focus on building the muscles that rowing does not address: mainly the upper body pressing muscles, including the chest, shoulders, and triceps, and the spinal erector muscles, including the erector spinae and the transversospinalis muscle group.

Pectoral Muscles

The pectoral muscles (pecs) are a group of skeletal muscles that connect your arms to your lateral and thoracic walls. They consist of the pectoralis major and pectoralis minor muscles, the serratus anterior, and the subclavius. They lie across the anterior part of our rib cage. The pec minor aids in scapular depression (pushing the shoulder blades down) and protraction (pulling the shoulder blades apart). The pec major attaches from the humerus (upper arm bone) to the clavicle (collarbone) and the sternum (the middle of the chest). The pec major has two heads: the clavicular head and the sternocostal. The clavicular head activates inflection of the shoulder and assists the sternocostal head to internally rotate and adduct the arm (pulling the arm toward the midline of the body). The pec major activates in the drive phase of the stroke (during the pull through the arms), assisting the lats. It is also a secondary muscle in the recovery phase, assisting the shoulders in flexion.

CHEST PRESS

INSTRUCTIONS

- Lie supine (on your back) with your knees bent and feet flat on the floor. If you're on a bench, your legs should be on either side of it, with your feet flat on the floor.
- With one dumbbell in each hand, extend your arms upward toward the ceiling *(a)*.
- Pressing into the floor or bench with your back, lower the weights to your chest, bending your elbows at a slight angle (not directly out to the side) and turning the palms of your hands at a slight angle toward one another *(b)*. If you're on a bench, do not let your elbows go beyond the height of your bench.
- Push the weights away from your chest back to the starting position, and repeat.

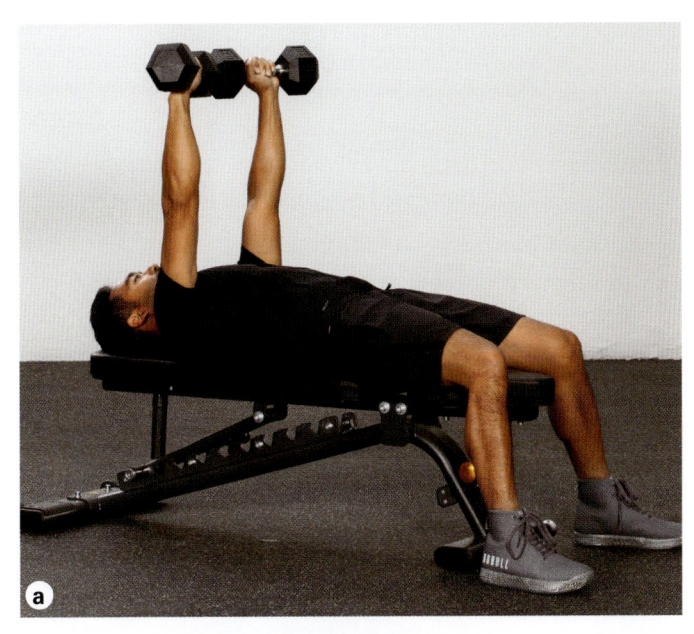

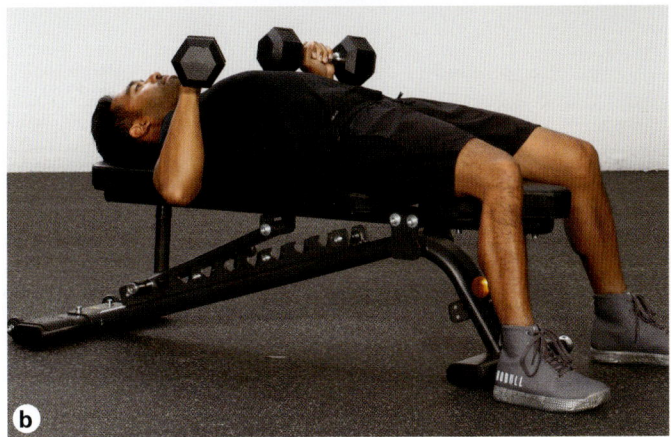

Off-the-Rower Strength Training for On-the-Rower Performance **139**

PUSH-UPS

INSTRUCTIONS

- Lie in a prone position (face down), with your hands just under your shoulders and your elbows bent and angled back (not directly out to the side).
- Tuck your toes and brace your core.
- Initiate the movement by pressing your hands against the floor to push your arms straight. Maintain a straight line from the crown of your head down to your heels.
- Bend your elbows to lower yourself to the starting position.

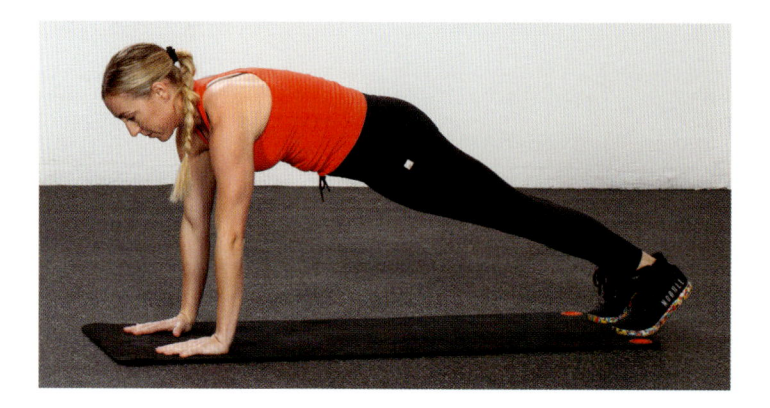

TIP To modify this movement, drop to your knees but keep a straight line from the crown of your head to your knees.

Shoulders

The shoulder's main motions are flexion, extension, abduction, adduction, and internal and external rotation. As a ball-and-socket joint, it is sensitive and prone to injury. The shoulder plays a secondary role in the rowing stroke when pushing the arm forward through the recovery. Internal and external rotation and adduction and abduction are not used on the rower. Secondary training keeps this joint strong and supported.

OVERHEAD PRESS

INSTRUCTIONS

- Stand with your feet shoulder-width apart, with a soft bend in your knees. Hold two dumbbells in either hand at a slight angle.
- Position the dumbbells on either shoulder and brace your core *(a)*.
- With a braced core, press the weights overhead *(b)*, pause for a moment, and slowly lower back to the starting position.

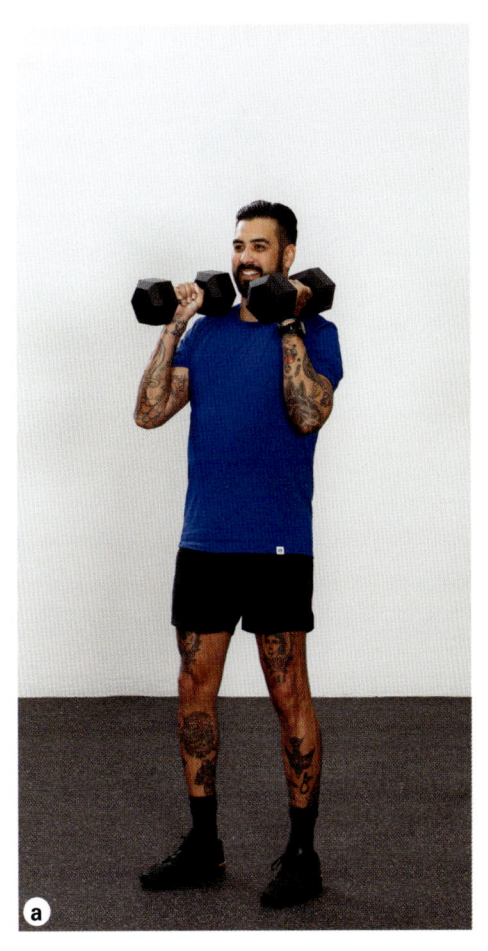

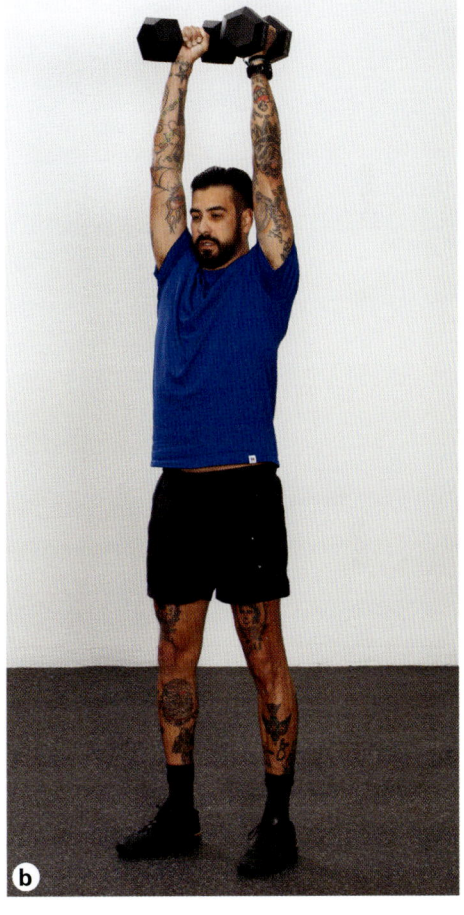

UPRIGHT ROW

INSTRUCTIONS

- Stand with your feet shoulder-width apart, chest up, and eyes focused forward.
- Hold the dumbbells in each hand and let them rest in front of your thighs *(a)*. You may also use a barbell for this movement; the barbell should rest in your hands in front of your thighs.
- Bend your elbows and lift the weights up toward your chin *(b)*. Pause at the top of the movement, then lower the barbell to the starting position.

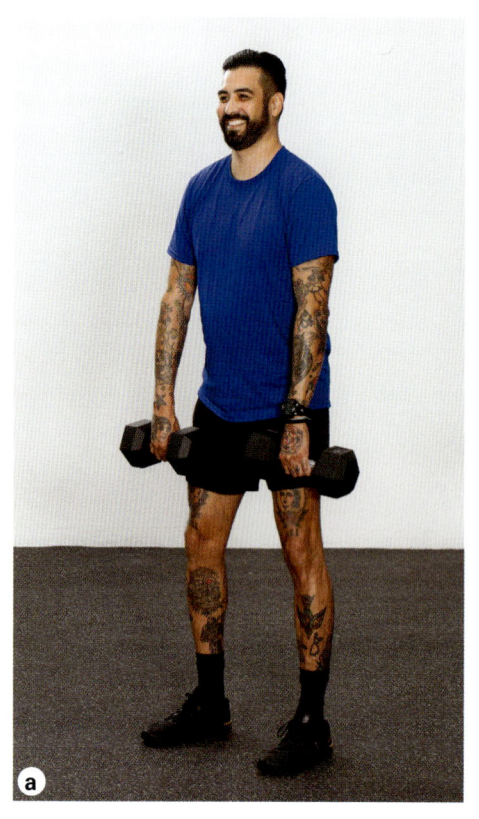

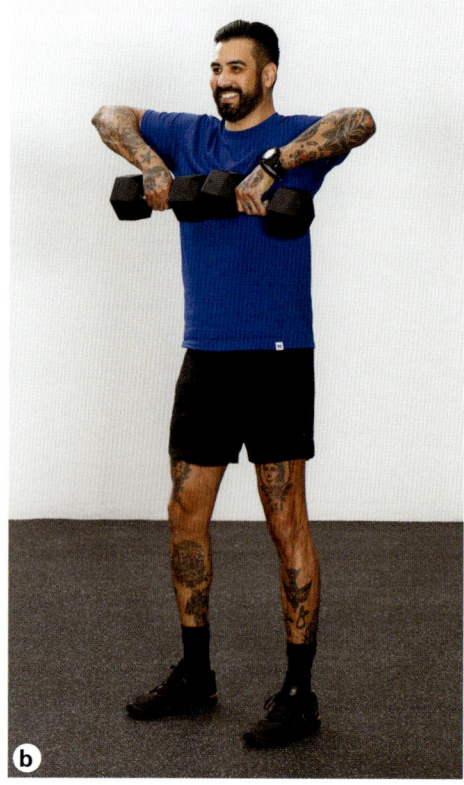

Triceps

The triceps brachii is a large, thick muscle on the back of the upper arm. The triceps' primary function is to extend the elbow joint. It assists in the extension of the arm through the recovery.

LYING TRICEPS EXTENSION

INSTRUCTIONS

- Lie on your back with your knees bent and a dumbbell in each hand.
- Extend your arms and position the weights directly over your shoulders.
- Bend your elbows and lower the dumbbells toward your ears, stopping when they are close to your ears. Pause and return to the starting position.

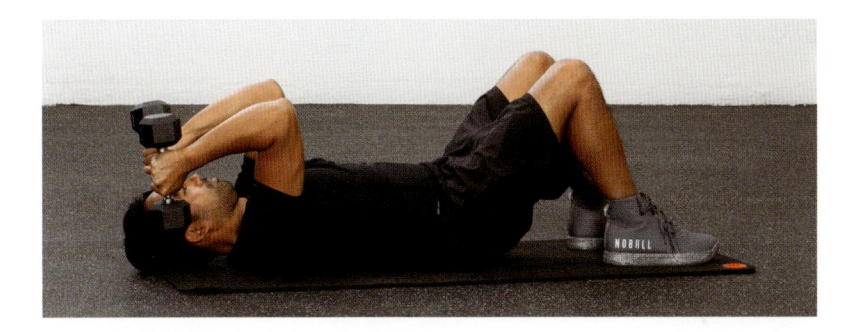

TRICEPS DIPS

INSTRUCTIONS

- Using a stable chair or bench, sit with your hands gripping the edge of the chair just beside your hips. Point your elbows to the back of the chair directly behind you.
- Lift yourself off the chair and slide forward so that your buttocks clear the chair. Extend your legs, keeping a slight bend in your knees *(a)*.
- Lower yourself until your elbows are bent to 90 degrees *(b)*. To modify the movement, perform a shallower bend. Push yourself back up slowly until your arms are straight, and repeat.

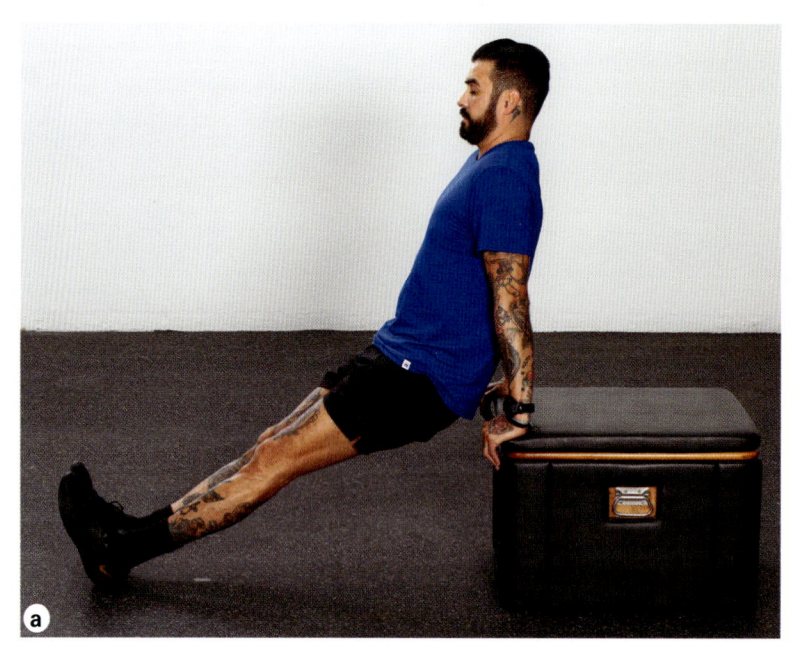

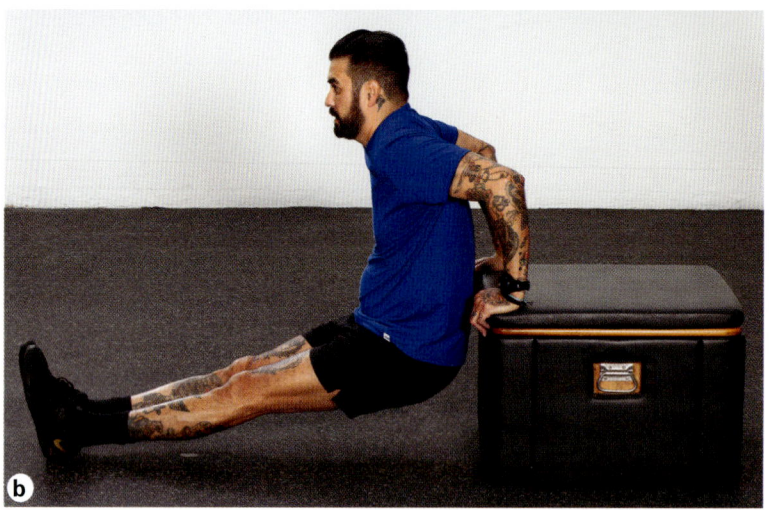

Spinal Erector Muscles

The spinal erector muscles, including the iliocostalis, longissimus, and spinalis, play an important role in the function and movement of the entire body. They run vertically down your entire back on either side of your spine and are superficial to larger muscles. They are responsible for keeping you upright and controlling forward flexion. Additionally, they aid in torso rotation and certain head movements. We'll focus here on two movements that will allow for strengthening these muscles.

SUPERMAN

INSTRUCTIONS

- Lie on the floor in a prone position (face down), with your legs straight and your arms extended in front of you.
- Keep your head in a neutral position and your belly button pulling toward the spine.
- Slowly lift your arms and legs about 6 inches (15.3 cm) off the floor, or until you feel your lower back muscles contract. Keep your abs engaged and lifted off the floor. Hold for 2 to 3 seconds, then lower to the starting position.
- Repeat for the desired number of repetitions.

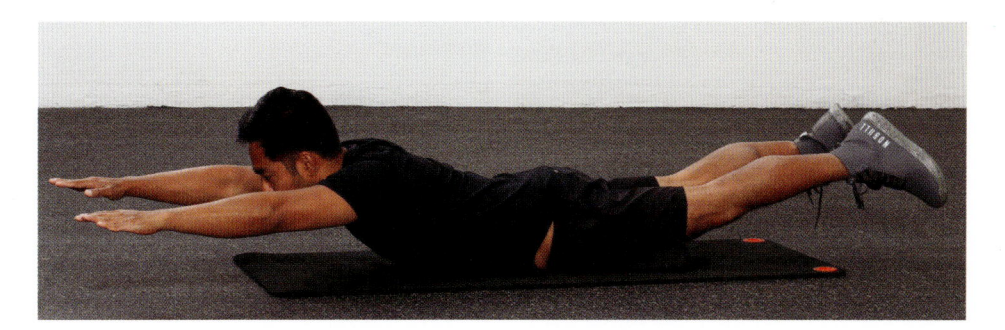

GOOD MORNINGS

INSTRUCTIONS

- Prepare a barbell on a squat rack.
- Step under the bar with your feet hip-distance apart and place the bar on your back, just above your shoulder blades *(a)*. Be careful not to place the bar on your neck. Brace your core to stabilize the lumbar spine and ensure that your spine is long.
- Begin the movement by hinging forward at the hips, controlling your torso as you lengthen slowly toward the floor. Keep your back straight, your neck neutral, and your gaze forward *(b)*. Allow your knees to bend. As your hamstrings lengthen, you will feel tightness, which is your cue that you've hinged far enough. Do NOT allow your back to flex.
- Return to standing, opening the hips and flexing the glutes. Repeat for the desired number of repetitions.

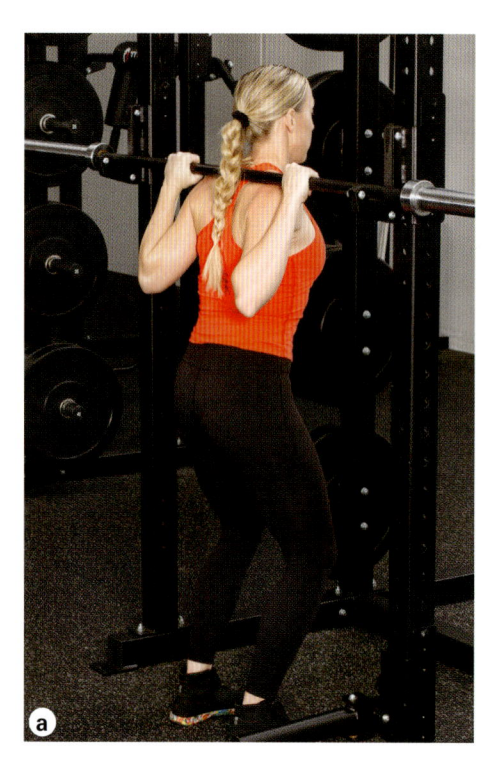

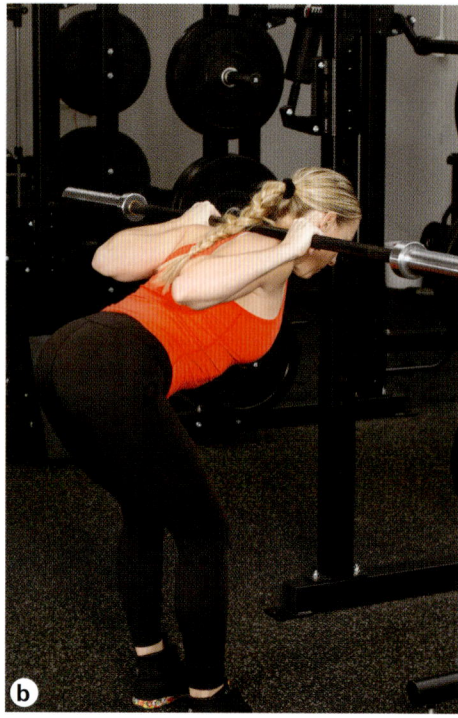

Developing key muscle groups such as the back, shoulders, arms, legs, and core will have an impact on your strength and power and how well you execute your movements on the rowing machine. Addressing muscular imbalances and promoting joint stability will help mitigate the risk of an overuse injury associated with the repetitive nature of the rowing stroke.

10

INCORPORATING ROWING INTO STRENGTH AND FITNESS ROUTINES

You have many options for working rowing into your current strength training or fitness routine. Whether you're just getting started in fitness, training for a marathon or triathlon, recovering from an injury, or simply looking to maintain an active lifestyle, rowing is a beneficial addition to your routine.

When deciding how to incorporate rowing into your training, the first step is to identify your goal by answering the following questions:

1. Is there an event or race you are training for? If so, what?
2. What is your goal, and what is your desired timeline to accomplish it?
3. What is your current fitness level?
4. How many times a week are you able to set aside time for exercise, and for how long?
5. Do you have any injuries or restrictions?

Let's look at each of these factors independently to determine how your answers affect the frequency and type of rowing workouts you consistently perform.

Is There an Event or Race You Are Training For? If So, What?

This question is important because, depending on whether you're training for a marathon, a triathlon, or a 2,000-meter or 500-meter rowing competition, you'll incorporate rowing differently into your workouts.

KEY POINT

Depending on what type of event you are training for, you'll incorporate rowing differently into your workouts. When you are assessing the best training method for a specific race or event, a great place to start is by considering how long the event takes and at what effort or intensity level you'll remain throughout the event.

For a 500-meter rowing competition, you'll want to train your anaerobic zones and boost your power output because you'll only be on the rower for a very short amount of time, anywhere from one to three minutes. Your body's ability to produce power on the machine quickly will be crucial to finding success in this specific benchmark or race. In order to maximize your power on the rowing machine, consider building more strength and power in your legs and core by adding some of the complementary exercises from chapter 9 to your workout routine. Movements like deadlifts and split squats are great for building strength, whereas movements like jump squats and skater lunges are great for building power. Shorter interval workouts in which you're sprinting for 20 to 60 seconds, or 100 to 250 meters at a time, will be good to train your body and mind in an uncomfortable state of maximum effort. You may also consider training with a variety of drag factors or damper settings to find your optimal placement. The 500-meter row is a maximum-effort, all-out sprint in which you will get to an anaerobic energy zone quickly. With shorter distances like this, every stroke counts. It'll be important to ensure you have a strong sprint start to get the flywheel moving quickly to build up momentum early in the race.

The 2,000-meter row typically takes most people anywhere from 6 to 10 minutes and is four times the distance of the 500-meter row. From a training perspective, you'll want to work to expand your lactate threshold and anaerobic capacity to allow for the additional time that you will spend working at maximum effort. Rowing interval repeats in the 500- to 1,000-meter range will be key to accomplishing a strong 2,000-meter row. You may also weave in some 2,000-meter row workouts to mimic the race event to practice your race plan and get your body ready for the longer, strategic sprint. Crew teams around the world use the 2,000-meter row as a measurement to determine whether athletes make the team and where they sit in the boat for a reason. It's much easier for athletes to power through a 500-meter race, and the difference in times is minor, whereas a two-kilometer row requires a higher threshold for cardiorespiratory and muscular conditioning, mental focus, and, quite frankly, a higher threshold for pain and suffering.

Shifting from highly anaerobic races or events to endurance events, let's look at preparing for a race like an Olympic triathlon or sprint triathlon.

For an event like a triathlon that doesn't have rowing but has swimming, biking, and running performed consecutively, you'll specifically need to have strong power in your legs for the bike and cardiorespiratory and muscular endurance for all three parts of the race. You can accomplish both power and endurance training for an event like this on the rowing machine in partnership with the traditional swimming, biking, and running training. The strength you can build in the push of your legs on the drive will directly correlate to more power in your riding during the bike portion of a triathlon. This is more important for a sprint triathlon as opposed to an Olympic triathlon because the sprint distance is half that of the Olympic. In a full triathlon, which includes a longer bike distance, you may rely less on leg power specifically and more on muscular endurance. How you incorporate rowing into your triathlon training will also depend on your body and what you need specifically to strengthen and prepare for your race. If your endurance is already strong, consider using the rower to build strength and power by incorporating a longer set of rowing intervals, perhaps even adjusting the drag factor or damper setting up or down throughout to mimic the feeling of adjusting bike gears in a race. You can incorporate this into your regular endurance training routine for the race. If you need to work on endurance, consider leveraging longer, more steady-state-type workouts on the rower to complement any other endurance training you're doing, whether swimming, biking, or running. The low-impact, full-body nature of rowing can be a great option to weave into your training because it is easy on the body, especially considering the high volume of running you may be doing.

For the full marathon run, you'll need to train your body for long-term endurance and stamina, as well as maintain a healthy body and joints as you train. We've seen many clients throughout the years leverage rowing as cross-training for their marathon preparation. Rowing is full body and low impact, which makes it a great workout to do alongside any longer runs you may have scheduled for training, because it will keep your body strength well rounded and is a bit easier on the joints than running. Rowing also requires a similar mental focus as running, which is a huge factor in a longer event like this.

What Is Your Goal, and What Is Your Desired Timeline to Accomplish It?

If you're looking to get in shape for a wedding, vacation, or special event, there is likely a timeline that will affect how you need to exercise. Whereas if you're looking to maintain or simply improve your overall health, you may not need to be as aggressive with your rowing training plan.

You may consider adding a higher volume of interval training to your workouts if you need to get in shape for a specific event in addition to building strength off the rower. A typical cadence for such a goal might be three interval and station-based workouts, one steady endurance workout, one pure strength workout, one recovery workout, and one rest day each week leading up to the wedding or special event. The interval workouts could be station based, blending rowing intervals with other off-the-rower exercises to build strength. These workouts, if designed well, might last 30 to 45 minutes each. The steady endurance workout would be a moderate cardio workout, maintaining above 50% max heart rate for at least 40 minutes. At least one workout each week that focuses purely on off-the-rower strength would be beneficial. Strength and muscle mass play a big role in how your body burns energy, or calories, in addition to how your body looks and feels. Finally, incorporating a recovery day with a light-effort row blended with off-the-rower stretches and core work would be important to maintain the overall health of your joints and muscles long term. And, of course, a rest day!

Depending on how much change you're looking to see and how much time you have, consider ramping up to this volume or even adding more volume depending on the circumstances. Additionally, if you're looking for real physical change in your body, you'll want to get a head start by giving yourself many months of training and consistency. Our bodies do not change overnight, and real change requires the discipline to stay consistent. If you're simply looking to maintain your current physical fitness status, you might consider a similar training plan that swaps one of the station-based interval workouts with a recovery workout or a rest day. Using the rower as a piece of your training allows you to also shorten the duration of your workouts due to the efficiency of the exercise. So, if your goal is to maintain your fitness level, a 30-minute workout that incorporates rowing may be plenty.

What Is Your Current Fitness Level?

Both intensity and volume will adjust depending on your current experience and fitness level. For someone who's just getting started on their fitness journey, the rowing workouts you incorporate into your routine can be shorter and more focused on building technique and foundational cardiorespiratory health. For an athlete looking to incorporate rowing into their routine, the volume and intensity of the workload can begin at a higher level. For instance, someone who's just getting started might begin with rowing pieces that max out at five-minute intervals, maintaining a lower stroke rate so you can learn proper ratio and timing in the stroke before increasing the stroke rate and heart rate. For a seasoned athlete, it might be fine to dive into a 40- to 60-minute workout incorporating the rower. A 10,000-meter (10K) row would be challenging for anyone, but for a seasoned athlete, it wouldn't necessarily put a dent in their training routine and recovery, whereas for someone new to fitness, it could be three days before they recover from a row that long. The three main factors that will adjust based on your fitness level are volume, intensity, and cadence.

How Many Times a Week Are You Able to Set Aside Time for Exercise, and for How Long?

Consistency is one of the biggest factors that affects your training effectiveness. Set yourself up for success by setting realistic goals in terms of how often you can prioritize your fitness. Do you have two to three times a week that you can exercise for an hour each, or four to five times a week where you only have 20 minutes? Both options can give results, but there will be a better approach depending on the time and cadence you're able to commit to. If you only have 20 minutes to exercise in a given day, you may benefit from a rowing-only workout where you get the heart rate up quickly and keep it up for the entire workout, while saving a few minutes to warm up and cool down. Intervals or even a higher-intensity steady row are a great option to maximize the results on the machine. Rowing is a great option because it efficiently works the majority of your muscles, accomplishing cardio and strength in one workout. If you have an hour to exercise, you can add a bit more variety as you incorporate rowing into your training. Perhaps you can find time to do longer, steady endurance rows with a proper warm-up and cool-down stretch, or work rowing intervals into a longer station-based workout.

> **KEY POINT**
> Set yourself up for success by setting realistic goals in terms of how often you can prioritize your fitness.

Do You Have Any Injuries or Restrictions?

Depending on the restrictions you have or injuries you may be working through, you'll want to adjust your training style and how you incorporate rowing into your workouts. As an example, if you're recovering from an ankle, knee, or hip injury, rowing can be great because it's low impact; however, consider shortening the stroke a bit to reduce the compression in your joints. The good news is you can still get a great workout while rowing with a three-fourths-stroke length; however, you need to ensure you're rowing properly to maximize the results as well as keep your body safe. The beauty of rowing with such injuries is that it mobilizes the joint without bearing weight or impact.

Another example might be if you're postpartum and recovering from a cesarean section and have medical clearance to begin an exercise program. The core strengthening aspect of rowing will be crucial for bringing your overall strength back so that you can perform your daily activities, such as picking up your baby or even just walking up the stairs.

For most injuries, it will be important to get clearance from your doctor before adding rowing or any exercise to your routine, and proper form and ramp-up time will be vital. Our suggestion is to ramp up the volume of rowing in your workouts and keep the weight light if you're pairing it with off-the-rower exercises.

A restriction might be something like pregnancy. In pregnancy, you'll also want to get clearance from your doctor. Your workouts may shift slightly to reduce volume and intensity. Rowing workouts where your heart rate stays at about 50% to 80% of your max is a good place to be, or within talking range. Throughout your workouts, simply make sure you're still able to talk and say fragmented sentences. If you can only squeak out one word at a time, your intensity is likely too high.

Table 10.1 outlines some of the primary goals that someone may have. If any of these are similar to your own goals, the actions shown on the right may give you some ideas about how to make rowing part of your own training program.

Rowing can provide results regardless of your fitness level or goals. While spending any time on the machine is a great first step, you'll be able to maximize your results by starting with clear goals and strategizing your workout program based off of those goals. As we dive into the next chapter, we'll provide a six-week rowing-based program to give you a kick start into your rowing journey.

TABLE 10.1 Specific Goal Training

Goal	Actions to reach that goal
Training for an endurance racing event	Train both your cardiorespiratory endurance and muscular endurance. Look to improve strength and activation in your slow-twitch (type I) muscle fibers. Form, consistency, efficiency, and mental focus are key strengths to develop in your rowing.
Training for a sprint racing event <10 minutes	Train your cardiorespiratory threshold and power output. Build strength in your fast-twitch (type II) muscle fibers. Ensure you're rowing well enough to recruit the most muscles effectively.
Coming back from an injury	Start slow and be intentional. Depending on the injury, consider focusing on mobility and stability in the joint. Avoid overcompensating on the uninjured side of the body by layering in unilateral movements. Unilateral movements allow for one side of your body to work at a time. In rowing, our legs and arms move bilaterally, which means both legs push at the same time and both arms pull at the same time. A recent injury to one leg, for example, may cause you to subconsciously push less hard on that side, which can create imbalances. Pairing your rowing workouts with unilateral strength and mobility exercises off the rower can be a great way to build back stability and strength in your injured muscle or joint. Keep it low impact by leveraging rowing as your primary form of cardiorespiratory exercise.
Just getting started in fitness	Build a strong foundation of movement! You are a blank slate, so proper form is key. Find an approach to training that allows your mind to find focus and feel empowered. Ensure you're rowing properly to gain the most benefit and results from your workout.
The aging body looking to stay fit	Keep it simple. Focus on improving bone density through strength training and cardiorespiratory strength with rowing, and top it off with mobility and flexibility work.
Lose weight and tone up	Build muscle, develop power, and burn fat with high-intensity intervals and consistency.
Improve heart health	Perform a blend of interval- and endurance-based cardiorespiratory rowing training.
Maintain current fitness level	Adopt a steady approach to training with challenging and achievable full-body workouts that maintain health and mobility in the joints, as well as build functional strength to improve everyday life.

11

SAMPLE SIX-WEEK ROWING PROGRAM

In this chapter, we've provided six weeks of unique rowing workouts to incorporate into your fitness routine. The program was built for anyone who's simply looking to add rowing to their fitness routine. Whether you are new to rowing or an experienced rower, this program can benefit you. You will also find some supplementary programs if you're looking for more volume. Because rowing machines have measurable metrics, we encourage you to keep track of your workouts so you can see progress over time.

For specifics on how many times per week to perform each workout, see detailed instructions listed before each week's workouts, including the number of workouts, how often and when to complete them, and the rest days, as well as specific warm-up and cool-down details listed within each workout.

Week 1: Laying the Foundation

When you start a new routine, especially one with a technical modality such as rowing, it is important to remember how building the best foundation will affect you moving forward. Be patient with yourself as you start to foster the mind–body connection needed to row well. The more you pay attention to the nuances of where your body is in each part of the stroke, the more quickly you will build those pathways to success! There are three workouts this week. Alternate the workdays with the rest days to allow your body time to acclimate to the rower. If you are new to working out or just restarting, you may want these to be your only workouts for the day. The goal would be to do all three workouts in week one, with one day of rest in between. If you are already on a workout schedule, you can incorporate these into your routine and do them on consecutive days, repeating the week's workouts if you like. Focus on technique starting with the fundamental hip hinge. The hip hinge is integral in a strong stroke and will protect your back from injury.

Week 1, Workout 1

This workout incorporates some of the key drills that will allow you to build a solid foundation in your stroke form. Take your time with the drills, and be mindful and aware of your body and how you're moving. The drills can improve your stroke greatly if you're executing them properly. A great method to ensure you're moving properly is to watch yourself in the mirror, if you have one.

This workout includes a short warm-up to allow the body to feel a proper hip hinge, then 24 minutes of rowing, followed by some final stretches. During the first few rowing drills, focus heavily on sitting tall in your seat. This will allow your hamstrings to stretch as you take each stroke, resulting in better body positioning at the catch and more muscle activation throughout the drive.

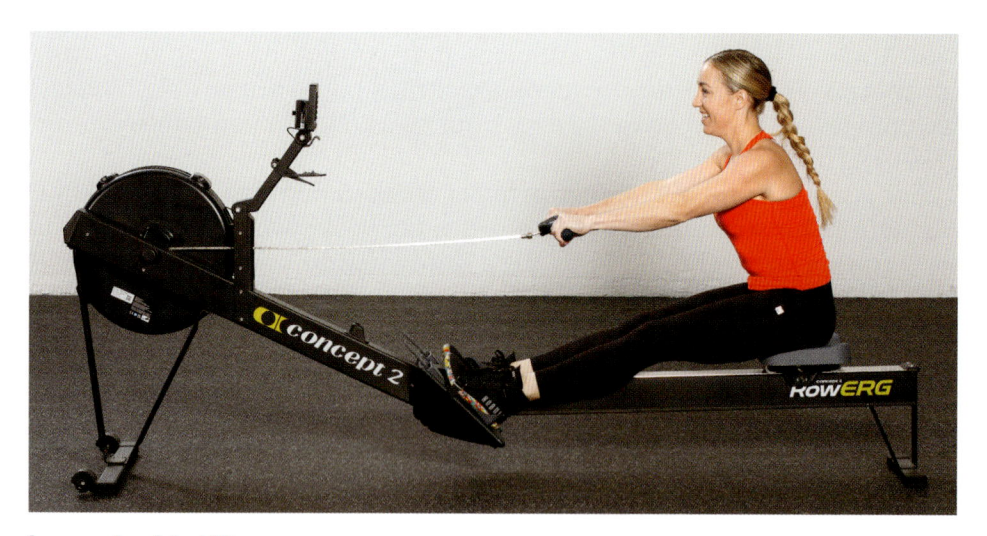

Legs only pick drill.

Week 1, Workout 1

Time	Drill or exercise	Page #	Stroke rate	Effort	Objective
2 minutes	Good mornings	p. 75	N/A	Warm-up	Practice the hip hinge, rowing's fundamental movement pattern.
4 minutes	Arms only pick drill	p. 96	18 s/m	Light	Work on the recovery sequence.
4 minutes	Body over pause drill	p. 43	16 s/m	Light	Improve the hip hinge and the recovery sequence.
4 minutes	Legs only pick drill	p. 98	18 s/m	Medium	Improve core connection and power generation.
4 minutes	Steady rowing	p. 111	20 s/m	Medium	Maintain consistency: Keep the stroke rate at 20 s/m and your split as consistent as possible.
4 minutes	Stroke rate ladder: up	N/A	60 seconds @ 22 s/m 60 seconds @ 24 s/m 60 seconds @ 26 s/m 60 seconds @ 28 s/m	Medium	Learn how to shift the stroke rate up while maintaining breath control.
4 minutes	Steady rowing	p. 111	24 s/m	Medium	Recover your breath from the ladder drill while working at a medium effort level.
4 minutes	Cool-down stretches	p. 103	N/A	Cool down	Pick four stretches that specifically target the hamstrings, glutes, quads, and hip flexors.

Week 1, Workout 2

We have added a few more minutes to your rowing workout today in an effort to slowly acclimate your body to being on the machine for a longer period. You'll notice this workout begins with rowing technique drills because they are vital to ensuring you're not only rowing safely but also learning to produce your maximal power and build efficiency. Do you think pro basketball players stop practicing free throws once they get to the pros? No way!

Week 1, Workout 2

Time	Drill or exercise	Page #	Stroke rate	Effort	Objective
4 minutes	Dynamic warm-up: Good mornings 4 rounds: 45 seconds work 15 seconds rest	p. 75	20-22 s/m	Light	Each round, focus on maintaining a braced core, spinal alignment, and true hinging from the hip joints. Feel the hamstrings lengthen as you hinge.
4 minutes	Arms only pick drill 60 seconds arms only 60 seconds arms and body swing 60 seconds half stroke 60 seconds full stroke	p. 96	18-20 s/m	Light	Focus entirely on form. Maintain a long spine as you hinge. Brace your core and use your legs to drive.
3 minutes	Body over pause drill: full stroke with 3-second pause, arms extended, body hinged forward	p. 43	16-18 s/m	Light	Ensure proper sequencing and positioning on the recovery.

Time	Drill or exercise	Page #	Stroke rate	Effort	Objective
5 minutes	Diminishing stroke rate ladder: up	N/A	2 minutes steady row @ 22 s/m 90 seconds steady row @ 24 s/m 60 seconds steady row @ 26 s/m 30 seconds steady row @ 28 s/m	Medium	Maintain consistency and find some intensity at this lower stroke rate. Remember the ratio: quick back, slow in. Focus on the recovery sequence: arms first, then the body, then the legs. For more information and direction on how to perform a ladder drill effectively, refer to chapter 7.
3 minutes	Steady rowing	p. 111	20 s/m	Light	Find control of your breath and build consistency in your rowing stroke.
10-15 minutes	Intervals 5 rounds: 250-meter row 1-minute rest	N/A	28-32 s/m	Hard	Find more power for these intervals. Get close to a 1:1 work-to-rest ratio
3 minutes	Cool-down row		18 s/m	Light	Recover your heart rate.
5 minutes	Cool-down stretches	p. 103	N/A	Light	Focus on stretching the hamstrings, glutes, quads, hip flexors, and abdominals.

Week 1, Workout 3

For this workout, you will measure your 500-meter and 1,000-meter times and compare them to where you finish in six weeks. It is important to benchmark your fitness so you can see progress. You'll notice this is the same workout from start to finish as the next time you benchmark your rowing. This is because you'll get the most accurate read of your progress if you keep consistent variables such as how you warm up, time recovered between benchmarks, et cetera. Remember, in rowing, milliseconds matter! Pushing hard on these benchmarks is key in getting the most accurate results.

Week 1, Workout 3

Time	Drill or exercise	Page #	Stroke rate	Effort	Objectives
3 minutes	Arms only pick drill	p. 96	20-22 s/m	Light	Focus on your hip hinge and control through the recovery.
3 minutes	Steady rowing	p. 111	24 s/m	Light to medium	
4 minutes	Dynamic stretches	p. 84 p. 75 p. 89	N/A	Light	60 seconds each: Standing hip cradles (each side) Hip hinge good mornings Squat stretch
12 minutes	12-minute power stroke EMOM (every minute on the minute): Perform 10 powerful strokes at the top of each minute. Recover with a light, low stroke rate row for the remaining time.	N/A	Minutes 1-3: 26 s/m Minutes 4-6: 28 s/m Minutes 7-9: 30 s/m Minutes 10-12: 32 s/m	Alternating light and hard	Maintain your timing (your ratio) as your stroke rate increases. The higher the stroke rate, the quicker the recovery. Keep the recovery slower and longer than the drive.
2 minutes	Sprint start practice: 1/2 stroke, 1/2 stroke, 3/4 stroke, full stroke	p. 117	32-40 s/m	Hard	This sprint start is crucial to starting a quick race like a 500-meter race.
3 minutes	Total rest				

Time	Drill or exercise	Page #	Stroke rate	Effort	Objectives
1-3 minutes	500-meter benchmark	N/A	N/A	Hard	If you're on a Concept2 rower, set the monitor to 500 meters to measure your exact completion time.
2 minutes	Recovery row		18 s/m	Light	Use this time to recover.
3 minutes	Total rest				
3-6 minutes	1,000-meter benchmark	N/A	N/A	Hard	If you're on a Concept2 rower, set the monitor to 1,000 meters to measure your exact completion time.
4 minutes	Recovery row		18 s/m	Light	Use this time to recover
5 minutes	Dynamic stretches	p. 89 p. 76 p. 78 p. 94	N/A	Light	60 seconds each: Squat stretch Walkouts Cat–cow Dynamic half pigeon (each side)

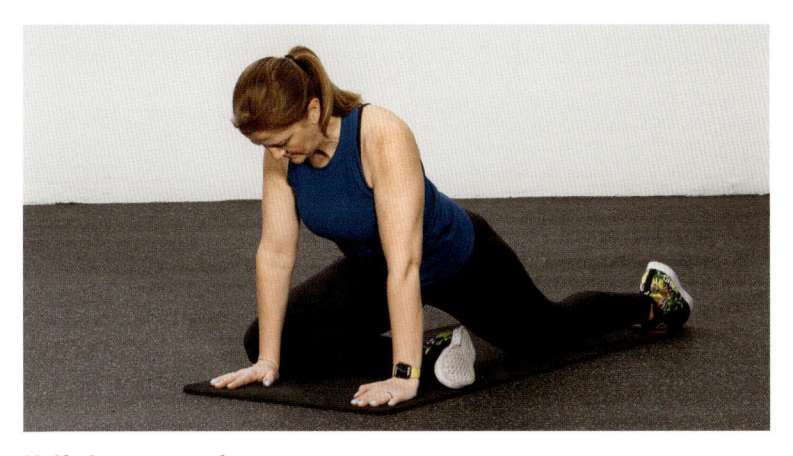

Half pigeon stretch.

Week 2: Building Intensity and Power

Week one is under your seat! Moving on to week two, our goal is to drill to find new intensities and stroke rates. It is very important to remember that there is an indirect relationship between stroke rate and split time. This means that you do not need to raise your stroke rate (move faster up and down the slide) to increase your intensity. Intensity comes from more "squeeze" or pressure in the legs. So you think about tightening your body and really putting force against the foot stretcher while bracing with your core to move the handle to the back of the machine.

There are only two workouts this week, each with their own focus. Do workouts 1 and 2 on back-to-back days, then take a day off and repeat them again. You can take two days in between if you feel you need additional rest.

Week 2, Workout 1

If you are new to rowing, this workout will allow you to begin testing the waters with new intensities and stroke rates. If you're not new to rowing, take this workout to the next level by being very intentional about your stroke rates and efforts. The stroke rate power stroke ladder will test your stroke control and your ability to build the momentum of the flywheel quickly. The sustained ladder will challenge your endurance. Be as consistent as possible with your split times; drop the split as you go up the ladder, and maintain the low split as you come back down.

Week 2, Workout 1

Time	Drill or exercise	Page #	Stroke rate	Effort	Objectives
8 minutes	Dynamic warm-up	p. 75 p. 76 p. 82 p. 84	N/A	Light	4 sets, 30 seconds each: Hip hinge good mornings Walkouts High plank to downward dog Standing hip cradles (each side)

Sample Six-Week Rowing Program

Time	Drill or exercise	Page #	Stroke rate	Effort	Objectives
11 minutes	Building power: Perform 10 powerful strokes at each stroke rate. Recover with 10 light strokes between sets.	N/A	20 s/m 22 s/m 24 s/m 26 s/m 28 s/m 30 s/m 28 s/m 26 s/m 24 s/m 22 s/m 20 s/m	Alternating light and hard	Develop an understanding of how to build power and resistance at any stroke rate. Recover for 10 light strokes between sets. Bring your stroke rate down to 20 s/m or lower.
3 minutes	Total rest				Allow your body to fully recover
11 minutes	Building control: Stroke rate ladder: up and down	N/A	60 seconds @ 20 s/m 60 seconds @ 22 s/m 60 seconds @ 24 s/m 60 seconds @ 26 s/m 60 seconds @ 28 s/m 60 seconds @ 30 s/m 60 seconds @ 28 s/m 60 seconds @ 26 s/m 60 seconds @ 24 s/m 60 seconds @ 22 s/m 60 seconds @ 20 s/m	Medium to hard	Start at a moderate intensity. As you build up in rate, drop the split 1-2 seconds with each shift. When you hit the 28 s/m on the way up, focus on controlling your breath. As you come down in stroke rate, maintain the split by adding power per stroke: quicker drive, longer recovery.
5 minutes	Cool-down row		20 s/m	Light	Steady row to allow the heart rate to come down, release lactic acid buildup, and refine your form and technique.
5 minutes	Cool-down stretches	p. 103	N/A	Light	Focus on stretching the hamstrings, glutes, quads, hip flexors, and abdominals.

Week 2, Workout 2

This workout will train you as a well-rounded athlete because the traditional rowing ladder drill begins with an aerobic endurance piece followed by an anaerobic interval piece. We start with the ladder to establish stroke and breath control. This ladder will allow the body to fully warm up prior to the high-intensity sprints. The final portion of this workout will allow you to find an anaerobic zone, which means without oxygen. Though you are getting a 1:1 work-to-rest ratio for the sprints and the rest is full rest, with each sprint, your body will need more and more recovery, and it won't get it. Not only will this train your anaerobic system, but it will also train your heart's ability to recover quickly.

Week 2, Workout 2

Time	Drill or exercise	Page #	Stroke rate	Effort	Objectives
8 minutes	Dynamic warm-up	p. 75 p. 76 p. 82 p. 84	N/A	Light	4 sets, 30 seconds each: Hip hinge good mornings Walkouts High plank to downward dog Standing hip cradles (each side)
11 minutes	Stroke rate ladder: up and down	N/A	60 seconds @ 20 s/m 60 seconds @ 22 s/m 60 seconds @ 24 s/m 60 seconds @ 26 s/m 60 seconds @ 28 s/m 60 seconds @ 30 s/m 60 seconds @ 28 s/m 60 seconds @ 26 s/m 60 seconds @ 24 s/m 60 seconds @ 22 s/m 60 seconds @ 20 s/m	Medium to hard	Start at a moderate intensity. As you build up in rate, drop the split 1-2 seconds with each shift. When you hit the 28 s/m on the way up, focus on controlling your breath. As you come down in stroke rate, maintain the split by adding power per stroke: quicker drive, longer recovery. For more information on how to execute a ladder up and down drill effectively, review chapter 7.

Time	Drill or exercise	Page #	Stroke rate	Effort	Objectives
4 minutes	Total rest				
20 minutes	Intervals: 10 sets: 60-second sprint 60-second rest	N/A	30 s/m	Hard	Make an endurance game out of this interval. Can you maintain the rate at 30 s/m for each round and keep your split exactly where you started on round 1? You can negative split throughout (rowing at a lower split) but don't let it go up!
5 minutes	Cool-down row		20 s/m	Light	Steady row to allow the heart rate to come down, release lactic acid buildup, and refine your form and technique.
5 minutes	Cool-down stretches	p. 103	N/A	Light	Focus on stretching the hamstrings, glutes, quads, hip flexors, and abdominals.

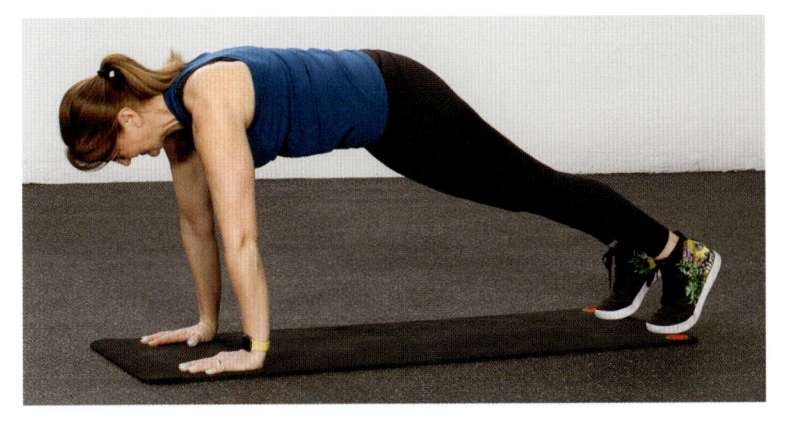

Walkout.

Week 3: Building Stamina

In week three, you'll start to increase the meters and focus on more endurance-based drills. This is going to help you understand what it takes to stay consistent on the rowing machine and put smooth effort into the machine for the most efficiency. There are only two workouts this week. You'll want to do them on consecutive days, taking one to two days of rest in between. You will repeat each workout twice.

Week 3, Workout 1

This ultimate ladder drill will not only train your cardiorespiratory endurance but also your mind. Be sure to take notes on your average splits and time for the first 1,000 and 2,000 meters, so you can try to beat your time and drop your average split as you come back down the ladder for the second attempt at these distances. Your effort on these pieces will likely sit between 75% and 85% of your maximum effort to maintain consistency and power throughout.

Week 3, Workout 1

Time	Drill or exercise	Page #	Stroke rate	Effort	Objectives
8 minutes	Dynamic warm-up	p. 91 p. 84 p. 88 p. 89	N/A	Light	4 sets, 30 seconds each: Hip rotations Standing hip cradles (each side) Tin soldiers Squat stretch
4 minutes	Arms Only Pick drill and steady rowing	p. 96 p. 111	20 s/m	Light	Do the pick drill (arms only, arms and body, half stroke, full stroke) for the first 2-3 minutes. Settle into a steady effort for the remaining time.
3-5 minutes	1,000-meter row	N/A	20 s/m	Medium to hard	Work at about 80%-85% effort.

Sample Six-Week Rowing Program

Time	Drill or exercise	Page #	Stroke rate	Effort	Objectives
1 minute	Total rest				Recover and record your time on the 1,000-meter row.
6-12 minutes	2,000-meter row	N/A	22 s/m	Medium to hard	Maintain or drop your split.
2 minutes	Total rest				Recover and record your time on the 2,000-meter row.
10-18 minutes	3,000-meter row	N/A	24 s/m	Medium	Maintain or drop your split.
3 minutes	Total rest				Recover and record your time on the 3,000-meter row.
6-12 minutes	2,000-meter row	N/A	26 s/m	Medium to hard	Focus on controlling your breath. Drop your split from the previous 2,000-meter row.
2 minutes	Total rest				Recover and record your time on the 2,000-meter row.
3-5 minutes	1,000-meter row	N/A	28 s/m	Hard	Focus on controlling your breath. Push the limits a bit on this one. Drop your split from the first 1,000-meter row.
3 minutes	Cool-down row		20 s/m	Light	Let the body and heart recover.
5 minutes	Cool-down stretches	p. 103	N/A	Light	Focus on stretching the hamstrings, glutes, quads, hip flexors, and abdominals.

Week 3, Workout 2

The ultimate ladder workout! This workout is designed to not only train your aerobic endurance but also your mental focus and control. Concentrate on controlling your breath and your split time. Try to be conservative as you begin the ladder piece so you can slowly drop your split as the rates and distances shift.

Week 3, Workout 2

Time	Drill or exercise	Page #	Stroke rate	Effort	Objectives
5 minutes	Dynamic warm-up: 5-minute AMRAP (as many rounds as possible): 5 walkouts 5 world's greatest stretch (each side)	p. 76 p. 92	N/A	Light	Move with intention and warm up the posterior chain, shoulders, and hips.
4 minutes	Double pause drill	p. 43	18 s/m	Light	Focus on maintaining a strong core connection and holding your body at 1:00 when you take your arms away to pause. Follow up with a strong hip hinge to pause.
3 minutes	Steady rowing	p. 111	22 s/m	Light	With light pressure (about 60% effort in the leg drive), focus on consistency in your timing (ratio: one-count drive, three-count recovery).

Time	Drill or exercise	Page #	Stroke rate	Effort	Objectives
N/A	Endurance training at different stroke rates	N/A	1,000 meters @ 18 s/m 900 meters @ 20 s/m (−1 second off split) 800 meters @ 22 s/m (−1 second off split) 700 meters @ 24 s/m (−1 second off split) 600 meters @ 26 s/m (−1 second off split) 500 meters @ 28 s/m (−1 second off split) 600 meters @ 26 s/m (maintain low split) 700 meters @ 24 s/m (maintain low split) 800 meters @ 22 s/m (maintain low split) 900 meters @ 20 s/m (maintain low split) 1000 meters @ 18 s/m (maintain low split)	Medium to hard	Control the split and focus on maintaining effort throughout. Note that there is no rest built into this workout. Start conservatively with your effort and build throughout.
3 minutes	Cool-down row		18 s/m	Light	With light pressure in the legs (50%-60% effort on the leg drive), start to bring your heart rate down while maintaining a strong core connection from the feet to fingertips.
5 minutes	Cool-down stretches	p. 103	N/A	Light	Focus on opening the hips, hamstrings, glutes, and abdominals.

Week 4: Intervals and Recovery Training

Recovery is critical for avoiding burnout and maintain high levels of performance. So this week has a recovery component to it. This week has three workouts that will take you through heart rate intervals. The final workout of the week will take you through an active recovery. You'll want to execute the following workouts: Day one: workout 1, day two: off day, day three: workout 2, day four: workout 3. You can repeat workouts 2 and 3 on days five and six if you want to do a six-day week.

Week 4, Workout 1

Workout 1 this week will introduce you to intervals on the rower! Have fun with this and really pay attention to what happens to your breath as you push hard, followed by rest periods. As you are rowing through the intervals, think of pushing to failure on the "on" efforts, and when resting for one minute, keep your legs moving but pull back on the pressure. Resist the urge to stop rowing all together. Teaching your heart to recover is a very critical piece of the puzzle if you're going to perform well for longer periods of time.

Week 4, Workout 1

Time	Drill or exercise	Page #	Stroke rate	Effort	Objectives
4 minutes	Dynamic stretches	N/A p. 89 p. 76 p. 78	N/A	Light	60 seconds each: Squat Squat stretch Walkouts Cat–cow
3 minutes	Arms only pick drill	p. 96	N/A	Light	Focus on the stroke sequencing
3 minutes	Legs only pick drill	p. 98	N/A	Light	Spend one minute on each part of the sequence: legs only, legs and body, full stroke. Focus on how the legs take 60% of the stroke, the body adds 30%, and the arms finish with 10%.

Time	Drill or exercise	Page #	Stroke rate	Effort	Objectives
10-16 minutes	Intervals: 100-meter row 1-minute rest 200-meter row 1-minute rest 300-meter row 1-minute rest 400-meter row 1-minute rest 500-meter row	N/A	28-34 s/m	Hard	These rowing efforts should be as close to maximum effort as you can give: aim for 90%-100% effort. As the distance increases, try to get your split back down to where it was on the previous piece.
3 minutes	Total rest				
10-16 minutes	Intervals: 500-meter row 1-minute rest 400-meter row 1-minute rest 300-meter row 1-minute rest 200-meter row 1-minute rest 100-meter row	N/A	28-34 s/m	Hard	These rowing efforts should be as close to maximum effort as you can give: aim for 90%-100% effort. As the distance decreases, try to lower your split with each round.
3 minutes	Cool-down row		18 s/m	Light	Focus on bringing your heart rate down. Holding your core connection between the feet and fingertips.
5 minutes	Cool-down stretches	p. 88 p. 89 p. 76 p. 92	N/A	Light	2 sets of 30 seconds of each: Tin soldiers Squat stretch Walkouts 1 set 60 seconds each: World's greatest stretch (each side)

Week 4, Workout 2

This workout is designed to challenge and train your recovery time. The work-to-rest ratio is 1:1 regarding distance, but considering you'll be working at a much lower effort and intensity on the recovery pieces, it will take you longer to get to that same distance. It will likely end up being close to a 1:1.5 ratio, which allows more time for you to recover. As the intervals progress, you may find you can't fully recover. Focus on maintaining your breath to help settle your heart rate during the recovery periods. It will also be important to keep the recovery rows' effort very light so you can maximize the recovery and give more effort to the powerful intervals. The good news is that the intervals will get shorter as you get more tired, so you should be able to maintain your effort and power throughout the workout.

Week 4, Workout 2

Time	Drill or exercise	Page #	Stroke rate	Effort	Objectives
4 minutes	Arms only pick drill	p. 96	20 s/m	Light	Focus on proper sequencing of the body on the recovery: arms, body, legs.
3 minutes	Legs only pick drill	p. 98	20 s/m	Light	Spend one minute on each part of the sequence: legs only, legs and body, full stroke. Focus on how the legs take 60% of the stroke, the body adds 30%, and the arms finish with 10%.
5 minutes	Dynamic stretches	p. 75　p. 84　p. 85　p. 86	N/A	Light	60 seconds each: Good mornings　Standing hip cradles (each side)　Inchworm　Hand release push-up

Sample Six-Week Rowing Program 175

Time	Drill or exercise	Page #	Stroke rate	Effort	Objectives
N/A	Vanishing intervals: 500-meter hard row 500-meter light row 450-meter hard row 450-meter light row 400-meter hard row 400-meter light row 350-meter hard row 350-meter light row 300-meter hard row 300-meter light row 250-meter hard row 250-meter light row 200-meter hard row 200-meter light row 150-meter hard row 150-meter light row 100-meter hard row 100-meter light row 50-meter hard row 50-meter light row	N/A	Hard row = 28-34 s/m Light row = 18-22 s/m	Alternating light and hard	Focus on training your body to recover as you row. Maintain your stroke technique from the hard row to the light row. For the hard row, drive hard through your legs and bring the rate up. For the light row, push lightly (while still maintaining muscular connection) on the drive and recover very slowly to regain control of your heart rate. Aim for around 90% effort for the hard rows and 30% for the light rows. Aim to get your split back down to the same number or lower on each hard-row round.
5 minutes	Cool-down stretches	p. 105 p. 76 p. 106 p. 78	N/A	Light	2 sets, 30 seconds each: Runners lunge + arm reach (each side) 1 set, 60 seconds each: Walkouts Down dog + hip shifts Cat–cow

Week 4, Workout 3

This workout will provide a full workout of active recovery training. Recovery training will keep your effort low and between 50% and 60% throughout the entire workout. Using endurance-based drills interspersed with stretching off the rowing machine, you will find warmth in the joints and muscles on the machine in order to find the deepest stretches off the machine. Your breath and finding length through the stroke will be your focus today. Length comes at lower stroke rates. Your breathing should never get to two breaths per stroke: an inhale on each recovery and an exhale on each drive.

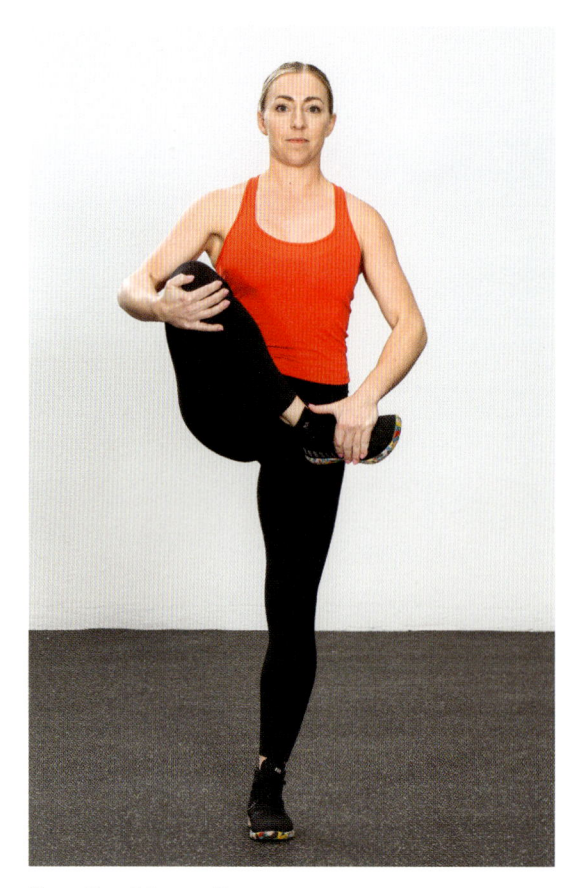

Standing hip cradle.

Week 4, Workout 3

Time	Drill or exercise	Page #	Stroke rate	Effort	Objectives
3 minutes	Arms only pick drill	p. 96	20 s/m	Light	Focus on the proper sequencing of the body on the recovery: arms, body, legs.
5 minutes	Steady rowing	p. 111	18 s/m	Light	Focus on your breathing.
5 minutes	Steady rowing	p. 111	20 s/m	Light	Pay attention to your breathing. Your split variance should be +/− 5-7 seconds, no more.
7 minutes	Dynamic stretches	p. 84 p. 89 p. 105 p. 89 p. 84	N/A	Light	60 seconds each (ladder style): Standing hip cradles (each side) Squat stretch Runners lunge + arm reach (each side) Squat stretch Standing hip cradles (each side)
10 minutes	Steady rowing	p. 111	18-20 s/m	Light	Focus on consistent light strokes, keeping your split time the same throughout.
6 minutes	Cool-down stretches	p. 76 p. 92 p. 106 p. 78	N/A	Light	2 sets, 30 seconds each, then 1 set, 60 seconds each: Walkouts World's greatest stretch (each side) Down dog + hip shifts Cat–cow

Week 5: Endurance and Mental Training

Learning how to row is a mental game! It's not merely a test of strength but also one of mental toughness to endure the monotony of the rhythmic motion of the rower. Because it is so endlessly challenging, the stronger you get, the stronger you can make your workout. Learning to embrace discomfort as you grow will train your ability, quiet your inner voice of doubt, and draw on what you know; good form and consistent effort will keep you strong. Your workouts this week will challenge your mental fortitude with longer steady rowing pieces. There are only two workouts this week but a lot of meters. You'll want to put two rest days between these and make them the only workouts you do on that day. You will fatigue, so go in prepared mentally and physically. Ensure that you are fueled properly for a long endurance effort.

Week 5, Workout 1

This workout is pure endurance training. Find an aerobic pace for the entirety of your 4,000-meter pieces at an effort you can maintain throughout.

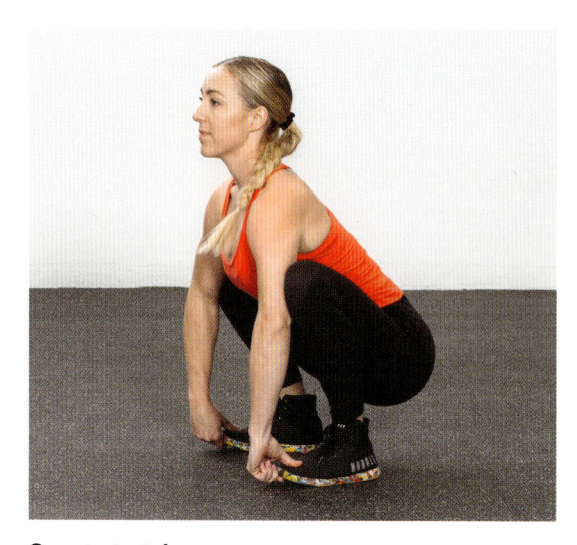

Squat stretch.

Week 5, Workout 1

Time	Drill or exercise	Page #	Stroke rate	Effort	Objectives
8 minutes	Dynamic warm-up: 4 sets, 30 seconds each: Hip hinge good mornings Tin soldiers Squat stretch Walkouts	p. 75 p. 88 p. 89 p. 76	N/A	Light	Focus on opening the posterior chain, or the back side of the body, to prep the legs and back for the rowing stroke.
14-25 minutes	4,000-meter steady rowing	N/A	22 s/m	Medium to hard	Use this first 4K to set the tone. Consistency is key. End just as strong as you started.
4 minutes	Total rest				
14-25 minutes	4,000-meter steady rowing		22 s/m	Medium to hard	Negative split −2 seconds from your previous 4K row. For this row, the average split should be 2 seconds lower when compared to the first 4K row.
4 minutes	Total rest				
14-25 minutes	4,000-meter steady rowing		22 s/m	Medium to hard	Negative split −2 seconds from your previous 4K row. For this row, the average split should be 4 seconds lower when compared to the first 4K row.
5 minutes	Cool-down stretches	p. 103	N/A	Light	Focus on stretching the hamstrings, glutes, quads, hip flexors, and abdominals.

Week 5, Workout 2

It's 10-kilometer day! The 10,000-meter row is a standard endurance-based benchmark and training distance in the rowing world. This 10,000-meter row will take you anywhere from 35 to 60 minutes depending on how low you can keep your split.

1:45 average split = 35 minutes
2:00 average split = 40 minutes
2:15 average split = 45 minutes
2:30 average split = 50 minutes
2:45 average split = 55 minutes
3:00 average split = 60 minutes

Be sure to record your time for your 10,000-meter row so you can retest and measure progress in the future.

Week 5, Workout 2

Time	Drill or exercise	Page #	Stroke rate	Effort	Objectives
8 minutes	Dynamic warm-up	p. 75 p. 76 p. 82 p. 84	N/A	Light	4 sets, 30 seconds each: Hip hinge good mornings Walkouts High plank to downward dog Standing hip cradles (each side)
5 minutes	Pick drill	p. 96	20 s/m	Light	Push back to the finish and hold. Start rowing with your arms only, add the body, then bend your knees and move halfway up the slide. Finish with a full stroke. Spend about 30-45 seconds in each segment of the stroke sequence.

Time	Drill or exercise	Page #	Stroke rate	Effort	Objectives
Varies	10,000-meter row	N/A	Rower's choice	Hard	Finish the 10K row as quickly as possible with consistency and good form. Maintain your stroke rate. Keep a low and consistent pace (split). Wait until the final 500 meters to let it all out.
10 minutes	Cool-down row and stretch	p. 84 p. 75 p. 105 p. 76 p. 107 p. 78	N/A	Light	Light steady row to allow the heart rate to come down. 60 seconds each: Standing hip cradles (each side) Good mornings Runners lunge + arm reach (each side) Walkouts Cobra stretch Cat–cow

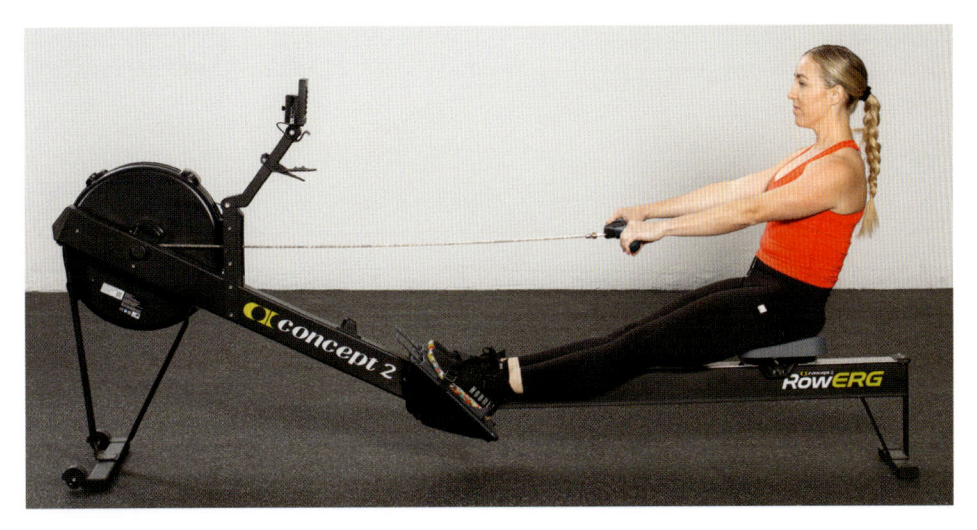

Pick drill.

Week 6: Benchmark and Recover

You made it to week six! Take a moment to congratulate yourself on all the hard work you have put in up to this point. This is a benchmark week. You've built your foundation and conditioning, and now you'll set your benchmark for the next quarter of your training. You'll repeat these benchmarks each quarter as a touchpoint for your growth. The goal is to drop your split on each benchmark!

Week 6, Workout 1

For this workout, you will measure your 500-meter and 1,000-meter times and compare them to where you started six weeks ago. You'll notice this is the same workout from start to finish as the previous time you benchmarked your rowing. This is because you'll get the most accurate reading of your progress if you keep consistent variables such as how you warm up, time recovered between benchmarks, and so on.

Week 6, Workout 1

Time	Drill or exercise	Page #	Stroke rate	Effort	Objectives
3 minutes	Arms only pick drill	p. 96	20-22 s/m	Light	Focus on the sequence of the stroke: legs, body, arms on the drive, and arms, body, legs on the recovery.
3 minutes	Steady rowing	p. 111	24 s/m	Light to medium	Consistency is key. How many strokes can you take without your stroke rate or split time changing?
5 minutes	Dynamic stretches	p. 88 p. 84 p. 105 p. 84 p. 88	N/A	Light	60 seconds each (ladder style): Tin soldiers Standing hip cradles (each side) Runners lunge + arm reach (each side) Standing hip cradles (each side) Tin soldiers

Time	Drill or exercise	Page #	Stroke rate	Effort	Objectives
11 minutes	11-minute power stroke EMOM: Perform 10 powerful strokes at the top of each minute. Recover with a light, low stroke rate row for the remaining time.	p. 118	Minutes 1-3: 26 s/m Minutes 4-6: 28 s/m Minutes 7-9: 30 s/m Minutes 10-12: 32 s/m	Alternating medium and hard	To keep the same stroke rate while dropping the split, lengthen out (slow down) the recovery right before your first powerful stroke.
2 minutes	Sprint start practice: 1/2 stroke, 1/2 stroke, 3/4 stroke, full stroke	p. 117	32-40 s/m	Hard	This sprint start is crucial to starting a quick race like a 500-meter race.
3 minutes	Total rest				
1-3 minutes	500-meter benchmark	N/A	N/A	Hard	Set your monitor to count down from 500 meters to measure your exact completion time.
2 minutes	Recovery row		18 s/m	Light	Focus on bringing your heart rate down.
3 minutes	Total rest				
3-6 minutes	1,000-meter benchmark	N/A	N/A	Hard	If you're on a Concept2 rower, set the monitor to 1,000 meters to measure your exact completion time.
4 minutes	Recovery row		18 s/m	Light	Focus on bringing down your heart rate.
5 minutes	Dynamic stretches	p. 76 p. 78 p. 106 p. 107 p. 80	N/A	Light	1 set 60 seconds each movement: Walkouts Cat–cow Downward dog + foot pedals Cobra stretch Child's pose

Week 6, Workout 2

This workout has a series of three different ladders with descending time spent at each rate. The ladder drill is a fantastic aerobic exercise that will not only improve stamina and endurance but also improve control and timing efficiencies in your stroke. This workout was designed to be an aerobic, active recovery, with the key word being *active*. This differs from your recovery week workout in that your effort will likely sit between 60% and 80%. Because the rowing machine is effort-based, you truly can make it what you want.

If you're looking for a little tougher workout, simply push harder and keep your 500-meter splits lower throughout. If you're wanting something more along the lines of a recovery workout, just lighten up the push of the legs and allow your 500-meter splits to sit a little higher.

Week 6, Workout 2

Time	Drill or exercise	Page #	Stroke rate	Effort	Objectives
3 minutes	Arms only pick drill	p. 96	20-22 s/m	Light	Focus on getting the arms away smoothly and following with the body before you bend your knees.
3 minutes	Body over pause drill	p. 43	18 s/m	Light to medium	Sit in the body over position, up and out of your hips. This will help trigger the hamstrings and glutes to activate. Push hard on the drive, then pause for 3 seconds in the body over position.
18 minutes	Stroke rate ladder: up and down	p. 100	3 minutes @ 20 s/m 3 minutes @ 22 s/m 3 minutes @ 24 s/m 3 minutes @ 26 s/m 3 minutes @ 24 s/m 3 minutes @ 22 s/m	Light to medium	Maintain light pressure for the 20-22 s/m rates. Add medium pressure for the 24-26 s/m rates. Focus on consistent, intentional movement and breath control.

Time	Drill or exercise	Page #	Stroke rate	Effort	Objectives
12 minutes	Stroke rate ladder: up and down		2 minutes @ 20 s/m 2 minutes @ 22 s/m 2 minutes @ 24 s/m 2 minutes @ 26 s/m 2 minutes @ 24 s/m 2 minutes @ 22 s/m	Light to medium	Maintain light for the 20-22 s/m rates. Add medium pressure for the 24-26 s/m rates. Focus on consistent, intentional movement and breath control.
7 minutes	Stroke rate ladder: up and down		1 minute @ 20 s/m 1 minute @ 22 s/m 1 minute @ 24 s/m 1 minute @ 26 s/m 1 minute @ 24 s/m 1 minute @ 22 s/m 1 minute @ 20 s/m	Light to medium	Maintain light pressure for the 20-22 s/m rates. Add medium pressure for the 24-26 s/m rates. Focus on consistent, intentional movement and breath control. Lighten up your pressure on the final 20 s/m.
3-5 minutes	Cool-down stretches	p. 78 p. 106 p. 94	N/A	Light	Timing of your choice: Cat–cow Downward dog Dynamic Half Pigeon (each side)

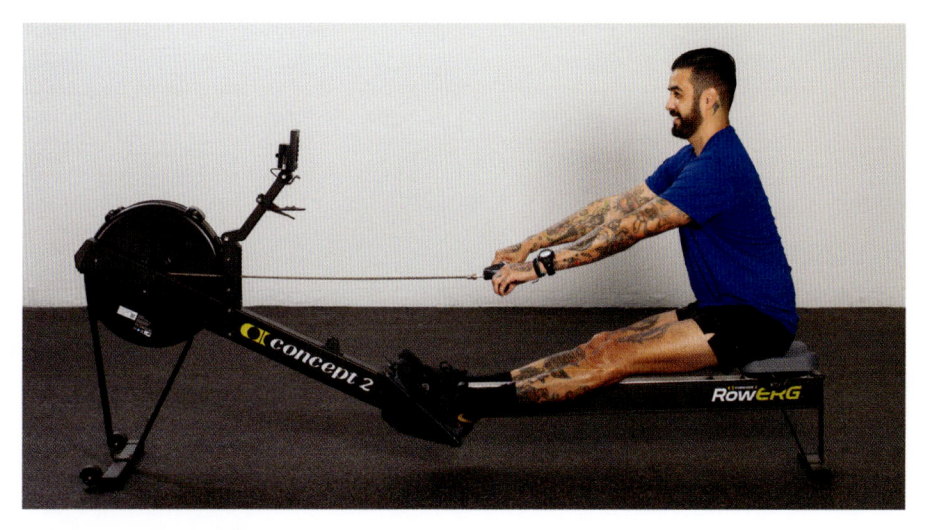

Body over pause drill.

Whether you are new to rowing or an experienced rower, integrating these six weeks of diverse rowing workouts into your fitness routine promises not only physical transformation but also enhanced endurance, strength, and overall cardiovascular health. By consistently challenging different muscle groups and varying intensity levels, you not only build a stronger body but also cultivate discipline and resilience. Moving forward, continue to leverage the versatility of rowing to maintain motivation and explore new challenges, ensuring your fitness journey remains dynamic and rewarding. Remember, the progress you made in these six weeks is just the beginning of a lifelong commitment to health and wellness through rowing.

REFERENCES

INTRODUCTION

Harvard Medical School. 2021. "Calories Burned in 30 Minutes for People of Three Different Weights." March 8, 2021. Harvard Health Publishing. www.health.harvard.edu/diet-and-weight-loss/calories-burned-in-30-minutes-for-people-of-three-different-weights.

Koch, T. 2018. "The Ancient Egyptian Rowing Stroke: Propelling the Boats of Gods and Men." March 2, 2018. https://heartheboatsing.com/2018/03/02/the-ancient-egyptian-rowing-stroke-propelling-the-boats-of-gods-and-men.

CHAPTER 1

American Sports & Fitness Association. n.d. "The Importance of Mobility for Aging Adults." Accessed March 26, 2024. www.americansportandfitness.com/blogs/fitness-blog/the-importance-of-mobility-for-aging-adults.

"Calories burned in 30-minute activities." Harvard Health Publishing. March 8, 2021. www.health.harvard.edu/diet-and-weight-loss/calories-burned-in-30-minutes-for-people-of-three-different-weights.

Castillo-Garzón M.J., J.R. Ruiz, F.B. Ortega, and A. Gutiérrez. 2006. "Anti-Aging Therapy Through Fitness Enhancement." *Clinical Interventions in Aging.* 1 (3): 213-20. https://doi.org10.2147/ciia.2006.1.3.213.

Chertoff, J. 2023. "Why Do Athletes Have a Lower Resting Heart Rate?" Last modified June 26, 2023. www.healthline.com/health/athlete-heart-rate#ideal-resting-rate.

Cleveland Clinic. 2022. "Heart Rate Recovery." Last reviewed July 18, 2022. https://my.clevelandclinic.org/health/articles/23490-heart-rate-recovery.

Corliss, J. 2021. "Aerobic Exercise Helps Hard-to-Treat High Blood Pressure." Harvard Health Publishing. November 1, 2021. www.health.harvard.edu/heart-health/aerobic-exercise-helps-hard-to-treat-high-blood-pressure.

Ferlinc, A., E. Fabiani, T. Velnar, and L. Gradisnik. 2019. "The Importance and Role of Proprioception in the Elderly: A Short Review." *Materia Socio-Medica*, 31 (3): 219-221. https://doi.org/10.5455/msm.2019.31.219-221.

Harvard Medical School. 2021. "Calories Burned in 30 Minutes for People of Three Different Weights." March 8, 2021. Harvard Health Publishing. www.health.harvard.edu/diet-and-weight-loss/calories-burned-in-30-minutes-for-people-of-three-different-weights.

Johns Hopkins Medicine. n.d.a. "3 Kinds of Exercise That Boost Heart Health." Accessed March 26, 2024. www.hopkinsmedicine.org/health/wellness-and-prevention/3-kinds-of-exercise-that-boost-heart-health.

Johns Hopkins Medicine. n.d.b. "Perimenopause." Accessed March 26, 2024. www.hopkinsmedicine.org/health/conditions-and-diseases/perimenopause.

Mayo Clinic Staff. 2024. "Exercise: A Drug-Free Approach to Lowering High Blood Pressure." February 20, 2024. www.mayoclinic.org/diseases-conditions/high-blood-pressure/in-depth/high-blood-pressure/art-20045206.

University of Colorado Hospital. 2003. "Training for Cardiovascular Fitness." August 2003. Reviewed November 2009. www.ucdenver.edu/docs/librariesprovider65/clinical-services/sports-medicine/training-for-cardiovascular-fitness.pdf.

VO2 Master. 2020. "Part 2: How the Body Uses Oxygen." December 1, 2020. https://vo2master.com/blog/how-the-body-uses-oxygen.

CHAPTER 2

Sybertz, A. 2022. "Understanding Your Peloton Row Metrics." Peloton: the Output. November 9, 2022. www.onepeloton.com/blog/understanding-your-peloton-row-metrics.

CHAPTER 3

Concept2. n.d. "How to Use Your PM5." Accessed March 27, 2024. www.concept2.com/support/monitors/pm5/how-to-use.

CHAPTER 9

Hunter G.R., G. Fisher, W.H. Neumeier, S.J. Carter, and E.P. Plaisance. 2015. "Exercise Training and Energy Expenditure Following Weight Loss." *Medicine and Science in Sports and Exercise*, 47 (9): 1950-1957. https://doi.org/10.1249/MSS.0000000000000622.

ABOUT THE AUTHORS

Caley Crawford is a retired Broadway performer with over a decade of experience in the fitness industry. She was a founding coach and director of training and experience for Row House, a boutique fitness concept. During her tenure, she played a crucial role in expanding Row House from a single location to 96 locations at its peak. Crawford was also instrumental in programming and coaching for the digital platforms Row House GO and Xponential+.

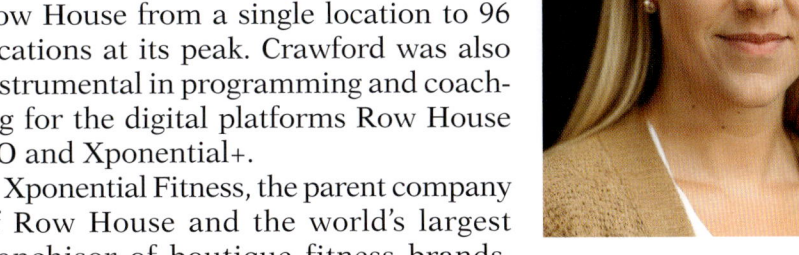

Xponential Fitness, the parent company of Row House and the world's largest franchisor of boutique fitness brands, announced in January 2023 that 6 of its 10 brands, including Row House, were ranked in *Entrepreneur*'s Franchise 500 list for 2023.

In addition to her work with Row House, Crawford has served as a Concept2 master trainer as well as the head of customer experience for Myrow, a digital fitness concept. Her connection to rowing is deeply personal, because it provided her with a safe and effective workout during her professional dancing and Broadway performances in New York City, as well as during her pregnancy. In 2024, Crawford launched a new dance and theater training facility in Houston, Texas, called Broadway Dance Lab, where she incorporates her knowledge of fitness into the dance program to ensure students are staying safe and building strength through their training as dancers and performers.

Crawford holds the Pre and Postnatal Fitness Specialist certification from American Fitness Professional & Associates (AFPA), is certified as a personal trainer by National Academy of Sports Medicine (NASM-CPT), and has earned the UCanRow2 rowing trainer certification. She is certified in CPR and AED. She has a BFA in musical theater and is an Actor's Equity member.

About the Authors

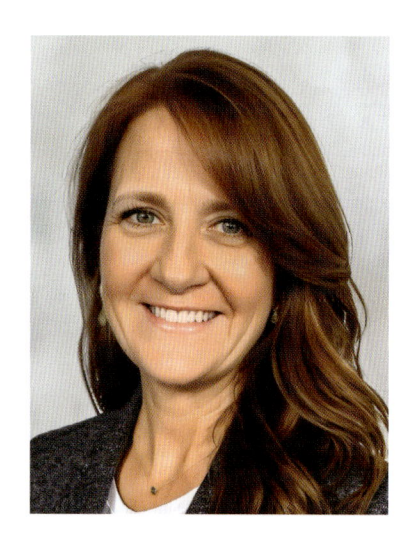

Michelle Parolini is a results-driven business and fitness expert with over 15 years of experience in managing coach training programs, developing leadership, and driving business growth in the fitness and retail industries.

Parolini was introduced to rowing at Row House Fitness as a lead coach for the first franchise location. She quickly grew into the role of senior master coach and the manager of coach development for the Row House brand.

Over the course of her time with Row House, Parolini has been integral in growing the brand and keeping their coaches up to date with the latest education. In addition to her role at Row House, she serves as a Concept2 master trainer and holds multiple certifications, including NASM CPT and Pilates Comprehensive. In her over 5,000 hours of one-on-one training, she has worked with LPGA, PGA, NHL, NFL, and Division I athletes, providing tailored fitness solutions.

Find more outstanding resources at

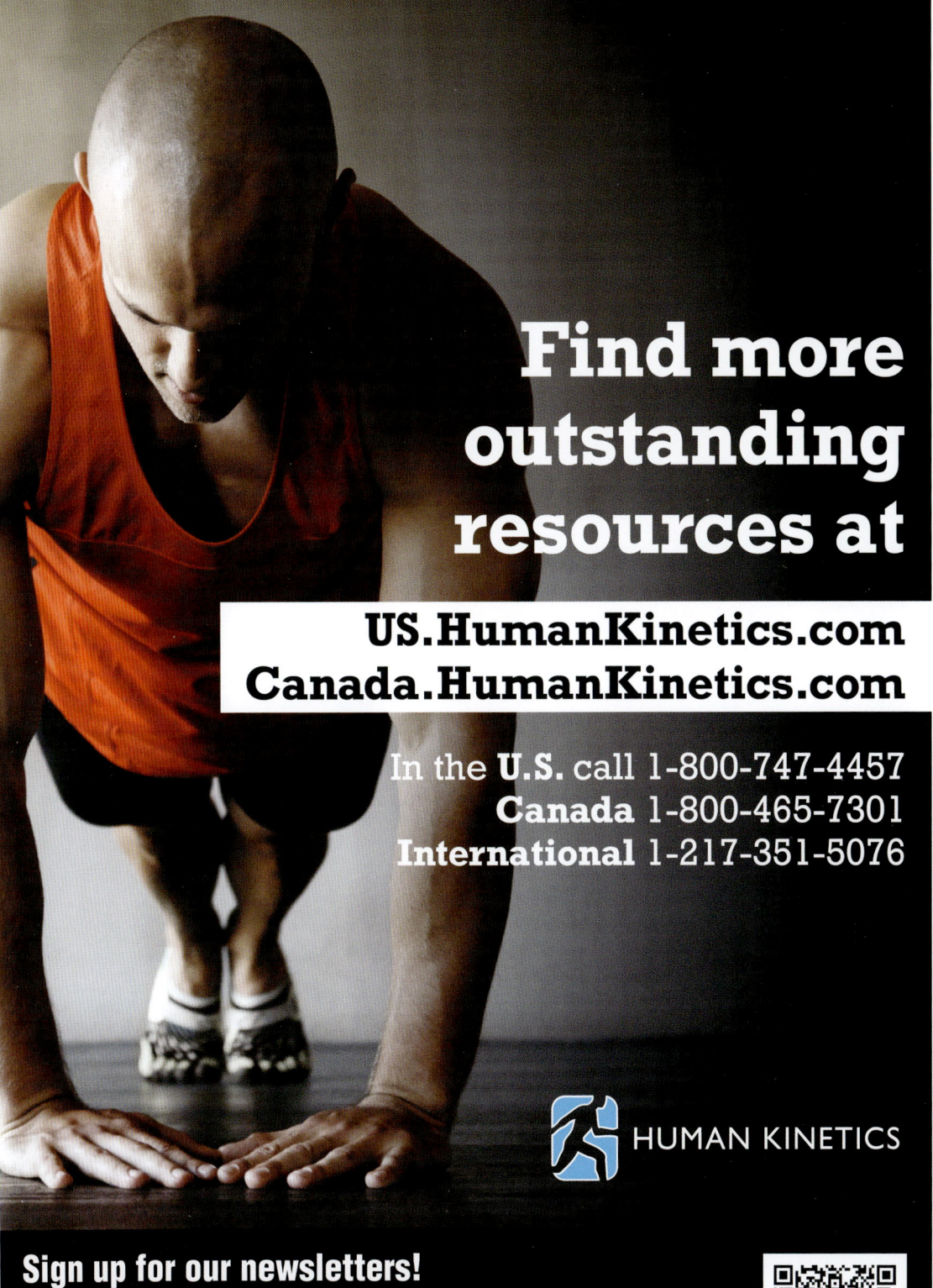

US.HumanKinetics.com
Canada.HumanKinetics.com

In the **U.S.** call 1-800-747-4457
Canada 1-800-465-7301
International 1-217-351-5076

HUMAN KINETICS

Sign up for our newsletters!

Get the latest insights with regular newsletters, plus periodic product information and special insider offers from Human Kinetics.

TAKE THE NEXT STEP

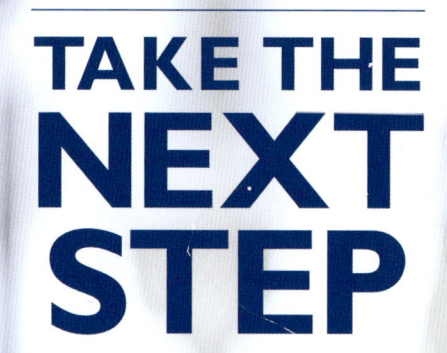

A continuing education exam is available for this text. Find out more.

NSCA
NATIONAL STRENGTH AND CONDITIONING ASSOCIATION

HUMAN KINETICS
CONTINUING EDUCATION

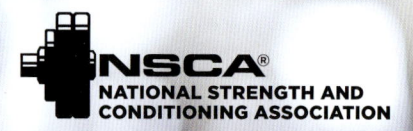

Special pricing for course components may be available. Contact us for more information.

US and International: US.HumanKinetics.com/collections/Continuing-Education
Canada: Canada.HumanKinetics.com/collections/Continuing-Education